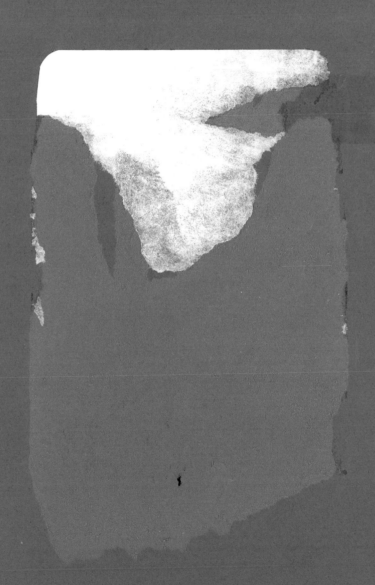

Female Sterilization

An Overview
With Emphasis on the Vaginal Route
and the
Organization of a Sterilization Program

Herbert P. Brown MD, FACOG
Clinical Associate Professor of Obstetrics and Gynecology
University of Texas Health Science Center
San Antonio, Texas

Stephan N. Schanzer MD, FACOG, FACS, FASCH
Clinical Professor of Obstetrics and Gynecology
University of Texas Health Science Center
San Antonio, Texas

John Wright • PSG Inc
Boston   Bristol   London
1982

Library of Congress Cataloging in Publication Data

Brown, Herbert P.
  Female sterilization.

  Bibliography: p.
  Includes index.
  1. Tubal sterilization.   2.   Vagina—Surgery.
3. Sterilization of women.   I.   Schanzer, Stephan N.,
1917-   . II. Title. [DNLM: 1. Sterilization,
Tubal. WP 660 B878f]
RG138.B78   618.1'059   81-16438
ISBN 0-88416-356-3   AACR2

Published by:
John Wright • PSG Inc, 545 Great Road, Littleton,
Massachusetts 01460, U.S.A.
John Wright & Sons Ltd, 42-44 Triangle West,
Bristol BS8 1EX, England

Medicine is an ever-changing science. As new research and clinical experience broaden
our knowledge, changes in treatment and drug therapy are required. The authors and
the publisher of this work have made every effort to ensure that the treatment and drug
dosage schedules herein are accurate and in accord with the standards accepted at the
time of publication. Readers are advised, however, to check the product information
sheet included in the package of each drug they plan to administer to be certain that
changes have not been made in the recommended dose or in the indications and contraindications for administration. This recommendation is of particular importance in
regard to new or infrequently used drugs.

Printed in Great Britain by John Wright & Sons (Printing) Ltd,
at the Stonebridge Press, Bristol

International Standard Book Number: 0-88416-356-3

Library of Congress Catalog Card Number: 81-16438

DEDICATION

Toward improving the quality of life.

To Sylvia and Kay for suffering the demands of a "jealous mistress," Medicine.

CONTENTS

FOREWORD

Doctors Brown and Schanzer have based this monograph upon their personal experiences with 500 tubal ligations performed via a transvaginal approach.

In addition to describing their own techniques, the authors have provided an excellent discussion of tubal sterilization in general. The monograph provides high quality coverage of all pertinent aspects of tubal sterilization, including alternatives to the transvaginal approach.

Chapter 5, dealing with preparation of the patient, and Chapter 6, which discusses medical-legal considerations, will be of particular value to many readers, because these chapters contain useful information which is seldom found in other source books.

The authors are to be congratulated for this excellent presentation.

Carl J. Pauerstein MD
Professor and Chairman
Department of Obstetrics and Gynecology
University of Texas Health Science Center

PREFACE

This monograph is based upon the personal experience of the authors with 500 colpoceliotomy Fallopian tubal sterilizations. This prospective study allows for drawing conclusions, biases, and recommendations, and proposes a detailed plan for interested clinicians to start a sterilization program or at least to give this method a fair try.

We wish to thank Mr. Emerson Bell, former Clinic Director of Reproductive Services; Ms. Mary Foster, Operating Room Supervisor at Park North General Hospital; Ms. Linda Bueno, critical typist; Dr. James Kurn, anesthesiologist, for providing excellent and safe anesthesia and for writing in part the section on anesthesia; and of course the federal and Texas state governments for providing the funds under the Titles XIX and XX of the Social Security Act.

Last, but not least, we wish to thank our patients who let us gain the experience with this method of sterilization upon which this monograph is based.

1 The Need for Sterilization: Past and Present

Man's wish to control his fertility dates back to time immemorial and many references to his attempts can be found in every civilization since recorded time. In his desire for reproductive choice can be seen not only his wish for personal comfort and pleasure but attempts to deal with the more central issues of poverty, ill health, and lack of education resulting from overpopulation.

Population dynamics and control are beyond the scope of this monograph but some pertinent data are useful to place the practice of sexual sterilization in perspective. Table 1-1 illustrates the geometric relationship between population growth and time.

Such staggering statistics emphasize the need for more and varied contraceptive methods. Of these, surgical sterilization has until recently been restricted because of legal, moral, religious, and social issues, and performed mostly for purely medical indications.

1

Table 1-1
World Population Expansion Rate by Time[1]

Date	Estimated World Population (billions)	Time for Population to Double (years)
8000 BC (beginning New Stone Age)	0.005	
		1,500
1650 AD	0.5	
		200
1850 AD	1.0	
		80
1930 AD	2.0	
		45
1975 AD	4.0	
?2000 AD		25-37

Furthermore, surgical sterilization was generally rejected by the medical profession because of its alleged association with a high morbidity and even mortality. In four major reviews of mortality statistics[2-5] from the United States, Canada, and England approximately five years ago, no deaths were reported in over 10,000 cases of tubal sterilizations. One study from India[6] reports three deaths from peritonitis in 2,269 cases (0.15%). Since 1978 there have been only twelve deaths reported in the United States associated with tubal "ligation."[7] These were based on reviews of hospital deaths and related to bowel burns, anesthetic accidents, and major blood vessel damage, all as a result of laparoscopically performed operations or associated with postpartum laparotomy tubal sterilization. *None* were associated with vaginally performed surgery, once again attesting to the relative safety of this approach.

It seems appropriate at this point to speak in more general terms. An operation should be undertaken only when the need for such surgery is greater than the risks involved. It would thus appear that vaginal tubal sterilization (VTS) performed by competent operators under appropriate safeguards is a justifiable procedure. Risk is inevitable, and in our society determination of safety is based on objective risk assessment, taking into account the above statistics, the normative subjective impact, and the social determination of risk acceptability. In Table 1-2 we have attempted to evaluate the risks of certain common life activities; we hope they

Table 1-2
Comparison of Risks*

Activity	Deaths/Person/Year
Motorcycling	1 : 50
Smoking (1 pack per day)	1 : 200
Horse racing	1 : 750
Automobile driving	1 : 6000
Being struck by automobile	1 : 20,000
Struck by falling aircraft (US)	1 : 10,000,000
Exposure to radioactive release from power station	1 : 10,000,000
Major surgery (hysterectomy)	1 : 1600
(other)	1 : 500
Using oral contraceptives (non-smoker)	1 : 62,000
Using oral contraceptives (smoker)	1 : 21,000
Using IUD	1 : 75,000
Sterilization (all types)	1 : 10,000 operations
Pregnancy	1 : 10,000
Abortion (less than 12 weeks)	1 : 50,000 operations
Abortion (more than 12 weeks)	1 : 5000 operations
Vasectomy	<1 : 100,000 operations
Leukemia	1 : 12,000
Influenza	1 : 5000

*Modified from Dinman,[8] Tietze,[9] and Center for Disease Control statistics.[10]

will serve as useful guidelines for comparing risks of known activities with those entailed in surgery.

It is no longer acceptable to consider death from childbirth as less objectionable than death from any other causes; the concept that death from a complication of pregnancy be considered an "honorable and inevitable event" must be rejected vehemently. Seen from this perspective, sterilization operations must be evaluated under the same terms as any other vaginal procedure.

As indicated in World Health Organization data, world population pressures have gradually produced a reevaluation of the constrictions against permanent contraception, leading to an acceptance of surgical sterilization as a safe, valid, and most effective

3

method of world-wide population control.[11] It is estimated that by 1985 more than 165 million people will have chosen sterilization as their method of choice. Table 11-3 illustrates world rates of use of the various family-planning methods.

Table 1-3
World-Wide Fertility Control of Women (in Millions) by Family Planning Methods[10]

Method	1970	1978
Voluntary sterilization	20	90
Oral contraceptives	30	55
Intrauterine devices	12	50
Condoms	25	35
Other (spermicides, diaphragm, sponges, injections, etc.)	60	30
Totals	147	260

The trend toward more permanent contraceptive methods is apparent; the table shows a four-fold increase in voluntary sterilization in the ten-year period from 1970 to 1980. During the same time span, an unexpected shift from primarily male operations to increasing numbers of female procedures has occurred. In 1970, of 942,000 sterilizations performed in the United States, 20% were done on women. By 1978, of an estimated 1,131,000 sterilizations, 59% were tubal sterilizations, a 3½-fold increase[12] in female sterilizations. During this same time the number of male sterilizations remained relatively stable.

Why should this have occurred? We have seen a remarkable development of assertiveness on the part of women in the last two decades as they have come to demand independent action and control over their own bodies. The chauvinistic requirement of husband-signed permission for tubal sterilization has finally been eliminated. The following conditions cited in Bonney's *Gynecologic Surgery* published in 1964[14] exemplify this restrictive atmosphere of the recent past and have well been laid to rest:

1. Both husband and wife must signify in writing that they agree to the performance of the operation and the method by which it is to be done.

2. The patient's general practitioner must signify his approval in writing.

3. The consultant in the disease for which the operation is indicated must also signify in writing that he advises the operation, eg, consultant cardiologist who should be a senior colleague of established reputation.

4. We feel that it is not fair to delegate this operation to juniors and it should be performed by a gynecologist of standing.

If these simple rules are followed no possible criticism can be leveled by the patient, her relatives, or her legal advisors.[14]

All of the above factors have led to an increasing demand for the availability of sterilization services.[15] The present monograph thus attempts to evaluate the currently popular methods of vaginal tubal sterilization (VTS) personally performed by the authors as part of developing a viable sterilization program.[16]

REFERENCES

1. Population Bulletin, 18 (1), Population Reference Bureau, Washington, DC, 1972, p 6.

2. Shepard MD: Female contraceptive sterilization. *Obstet Gynecol Surv* 29:739, 1974.

3. Yutzpe AA: A review of 1035 tubal sterilizations by posterior colpotomy under local anesthesia or by laparoscopy. *J Reprod Med* 13:106, 1974.

4. Hughes G, Liston WS: Comparison between laparoscopic sterilization and tubal ligation. *Br Med J* 3:637, 1975.

5. Brenner WE, Edelman DA: Permanent sterilization through a posterior colpotomy, *Int J Obstet Gynecol* 14:46, 1976.

6. Sonnawallah RP: Vaginal sterilization. Presented at Second International Conference on Voluntary Sterilization. Geneva, February 1973.

7. Peterson H: Sterilization mortality surveillance. Presented at Association of Planned Parenthood Physicians Annual Meeting. Denver, October 1980.

8. Dinman BD: The reality and acceptance of risk. *JAMA* 244:1226, 1980.

9. Tietze C: New estimates of mortality associated with fertility control. *Fam Plann Perspect* 9:74, 1977.

10. Final Mortality Statistics U.S. 1976-78, Center for Communicable Disease Control, Abortion Mortality Surveillance, Atlanta, 1976-78.

11. Potts M, Speidel JJ, Kessel E: Relative risks of various means of fertility control when used in less developed countries, in Vumbarco BJ (ed): *Population Reports, M/F Sterilization, Special Topic Monographs* No. 2, March 1978, p M-57.

12. Green GP, Ravenholt RT: in Lubell I, Frischer MS, (eds): Does minilaparotomy for sterilization have a place in your practice? *Contemp Obstet Gynecol* 14:39, 1979.

13. Ibid.: Association for Voluntary Sterilization estimates in Lubell and Frischer.

14. Macleod D, Howkins J (eds): *Bonney's Gynecologic Surgery*. New York, Harper & Row, Hoeber Medical Division, 1964, p 528.

15. Op.cit. Lubell and Frischer.

16. Planned Parenthood Association and Reproductive Services, Inc, San Antonio, Texas.

2 The Development of an Approach to Sterilization

FACTORS LEADING TO THE CHOICE OF THE SURGICAL PROCEDURE

At present, laparoscopic tubal sterilization is the second most often performed gynecologic operation in America (abortion being number one). In 1978 an estimated 1,131,000 tubal sterilizations were performed in the United States, 92% of which were done by private physicians.[1] This is probably the result of laparoscopic services being offered primarily in areas of high population densities, which of course attract the physician-specialist. Physicians also seem to have a certain fascination with new and sophisticated technological equipment. This was nicely illustrated in a recent response by one of North America's outstanding laparoscopists: "I just love to do laparoscopy."[2,3]

7

In the case of laparoscopic tubal sterilization this enchantment seems to have persisted longer than is the usual case; however, the first wave of enthusiasm has slowly given way to a more thoughtful consideration of alternate methods.[4,5] The demand for sterilization operations does not exist only in large cities. Most of the smaller suburban and rural facilities in this country as well as those in developing nations may not be able to afford the expensive and difficult-to-maintain equipment necessary for the laparoscopic approach or have the services of a highly trained gynecologic laparoscopist available. In these settings a simpler, more readily available day-surgery method must be chosen. About 50% of the patients in the United States in the years 1970 to 1975 had tubal sterilizations done in hospitals with a bed capacity of 300 or less.[6] Many of these procedures were performed at the time of laparotomy or cesarean section; other patients had to be referred to centers where laparoscopic equipment and trained physicians were available. VTS and possibly mini-laparotomy would seem to be ideally suited to these smaller facilities where standard instruments are usually available and where gynecologists, general surgeons, and trained family practitioners routinely practice.

In the selection of a suitable method of tubal sterilization under such circumstances, the physician should consider the already available standard instruments and equipment in the standard operating theater. There, ancillary personnel can easily be trained to set up for day surgery (ie, outpatient surgery during usual working hours). The physicians need not learn to use complex and unfamiliar equipment or go through the prolonged training mandatory to perform safe laparoscopic tubal sterilization. The standard instruments familiar to him or her from daily gynecologic surgery practice serve admirably for VTS. Furthermore, only standard general anesthesia and usual patient positioning are needed; no potentially hazardous techniques are required such as steep Trendelenburg posture or hyperventilation to prevent carbon dioxide-induced hypercarbia.

Patient acceptance is high. The woman spends only a few hours in the hospital or day-surgery facility and can resume her normal activities in a short time. There are no visible scars, not even Band-Aids. Menstrual function is not altered nor is sexual activity influenced after the first two weeks (to allow for vaginal wall healing). Complications are rare and usually minor. The often feared higher infection rate with vaginal surgery has not been a significant problem in this or in other recently cited series.[7]

Suffice it to say that a segment of the fallopian tube should be available for gross or microscopic inspection, a not unimportant aspect in this litigational society.

In Table 2-1 a summary of selection criteria is presented.

Table 2-1
Criteria for Choice of Sterilization Procedure

1. Optimum utilization of hospital and physician time.
2. Well tolerated by the patient, allowing for rapid resumption of normal activities.
3. Performable in standard operating room with standard gynecologic instruments; expensive or hard-to-maintain equipment not necessary.
4. Suitable to outpatient, day-surgery facilities and working hours.
5. Easily learned and perfected by any gynecologic surgeon, without the need for special training.
6. Amenable to standard forms of general anesthesia; special anesthesia techniques or body positioning unnecessary.
7. Leaves no visible scar.
8. Has few and relatively minor complications.
9. Does not interfere with menstrual and sexual function.
10. Makes available tissue specimens for pathological examination of fallopian tubes.

CRITERIA FOR SELECTION OF A METHOD OF TUBAL CLOSURE

Having selected the appropriate route to the fallopian tubes, a further decision must be made: the proper method of occluding the tube. The selection should be based on simplicity and a minimum of tissue dissection, destruction, and manipulation. The chosen procedure should be applicable to all avenues of approach to the tubes; damages to adjacent structures, such as bowel burns or lacerations, should be avoided; bleeding and hematoma formation should be minimized; the operation should prevent or at least minimize future pregnancies in an isolated segment of tube in the case of tuboperitoneal fistula formation.

Table 2-2 summarizes the various methods of tubal closure, which may be categorized into seven main techniques: simple ligation; ligation and resection; ligation, division, and burial; ligation, resection, and burial; fulguration; clipping; and banding. The normal utero-tubo-ovarian relationships are diagrammed in Figure 2-1 for orientation (Figure 2-1).

Table 2-2
Comparison of Tubal Occlusion Methods in Common Use*

Method	Year of Introduction	Possible Approaches	Reported Failure Rate (%)
Ligation only			
Simple ligation	1880**	ML,LTY,V	20
Madlener	1919	ML,LTY,V	0.3-2.0
Ligation and resection			
Salpingectomy	1898	ML,LTY	0-1.9
Pomeroy	1930	ML,LTY,LSY,V	0-0.4 (2.5-5.0 at c/section)
Fimbriectomy (Kroener)	1935	ML,LTY,V	0 (higher when done postpartum)
Ligation, division, and burial			
Irving	1924	ML,LTY	0
Ligation, resection, and burial			
Uchida	1945	ML,LTY	0
Fulguration	1937	LSY(1944)	0
Clipping (spring loaded)	1972	ML,LTY,LSY,V	0.2-0.6
Banding	1973	ML,LTY,LSY,V	0.3

*Modified from Wortman[7]
Approach Code: ML = mini-laparotomy, LSY = laparoscopy, LTY = laparotomy, V = vaginal
**First American Voluntary Female Sterilization described by SS Lundgren, Toledo, Ohio, May 22, 1880.

From these comparative data it is apparent that, with the exception of simple ligation of the tubes without resection or division, all methods seem to be nearly equally effective in preventing future pregnancies. Yet, the variety of tubal occlusive methods in use attests to the lack of universal acceptance of one optimal method. The final selection of method is thus based on ease and safety of application, on the route of approach to the tubes, on the expertise of the operator, and on the availability of equipment and facilities. In addition, the method most commonly used in a specific locale tends to become the model for others to follow.

A brief description of the common techniques of tubal closure, their advantages and disadvantages, is presented, showing the advantage of our method of choice, the Kroener method, most suited for the vaginal route.

Ligation Only

Simple Ligation First proposed by Lungren in 1881,[8] this technique employs the use of a single, nonabsorbable simple ligature placed about the distal portion of the fallopian tube without resection or amputation. Because of the reportedly high failure rate, this method has largely been abandoned.

Madlener Technique Described by Madlener in 1919,[9] this method aims to reduce the risk of attendant bleeding, yet allows for

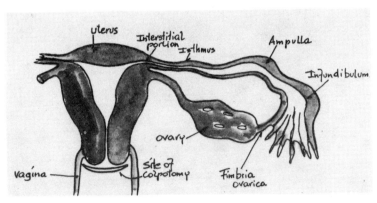

Figure 2-1 Utero-ovarian anatomy

greater ease of operation. The midportion of the tube is mobilized into a loop form, crushed across the base with a clamp, and free-tied with a nonabsorbable suture. Because of the relatively high rate of tuboperitoneal fistula formation, some clinicians perform a modification of this method where the loop is amputated, allegedly avoiding potential luminal reanastomosis, endosalpingeal regeneration, or tuboperitoneal fistula formation (Figure 2-3).

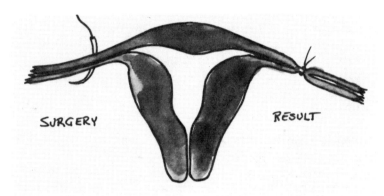

Figure 2-2 Simple ligation

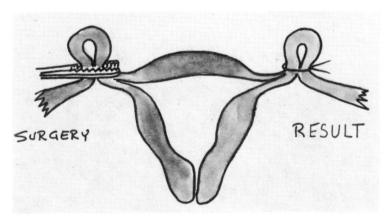

Figure 2-3 The Madlener ligation

12

Ligation and Resection

Salpingectomy   In this method the tube is resected distal to a nonabsorbable suture ligature placed around the proximal portion of the tube.[10,11] Because of bleeding from the mesosalpinx, this technique is not often employed (Figure 2-4).

Pomeroy Technique   This is probably the method of tubal closure most frequently used today. The description of this technique was only published after the author's death.[12] A loop of tube is raised near its midportion; the base is free-tied or suture-ligated with absorbable suture and a segment of the loop resected. Effectiveness of this method depends on the ready absorption of the suture material, allowing the obliterated ends to pull far apart, thus avoiding luminal reanastomosis or canalization. If performed as part of a concomitant cesarean section, a slightly higher failure rate is reported.[13,14] This method is popular because of its universal applicability, ease of procedure, and low failure rate (Figure 2-5). (See also Figures 9-7 and 9-9).

Fimbriectomy (Kroener)   Although originally used in 1935 with a six-year failure-free follow-up, this method was first described in 1969 by W.F. Kroener, Jr., the son of the original surgeon.[14] Tubal occlusion is accomplished by ligature of the tubal infundibulum with double silk ligatures and resection of the fimbriated end of the tube, care being taken to include the fimbria

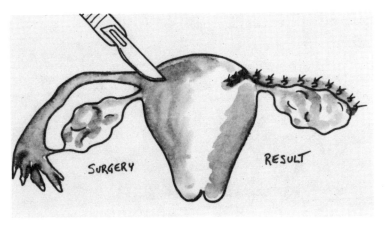

Figure 2-4   Simple salpingectomy

ovarica (Figure 2-6. See also Figures 9-5, 9-6, and 9-8). The advantages of this method are universal applicability, ease of technique, low failure rate, and minimal interference with the neurovascular plexus of the ovary. It is ideally suited to the vaginal approach.

Ligation, Division, and Burial

Irving   This method has a high effectiveness rate. As originally reported in 1924,[15] the tubes are divided in their midsection between two absorbable ligatures and the proximal stump

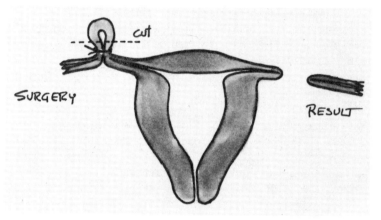

Figure 2-5   The Pomeroy segmental resection

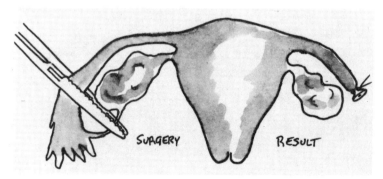

Figure 2-6   Kroener fimbriectomy

14

buried in the posterior-fundal myometrium. A high rate of attendant bleeding and the complexity of the procedure limit it to the open laparotomy approach (Figure 2-7).

Uchida   Developed in the mid-forties in Japan, this method was not reported until 1975,[16] as part of a mini-laparotomy program. A bleb is raised beneath the tubal serosa, exposing the ampullary portion where the tube is severed; both ends are tied with nonabsorbable suture; a 5-cm denuded proximal portion is resected; the serosa is purse-stringed over the proximal stump; and

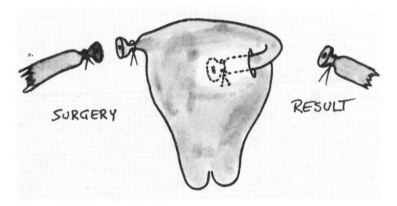

Figure 2-7   The Irving operation

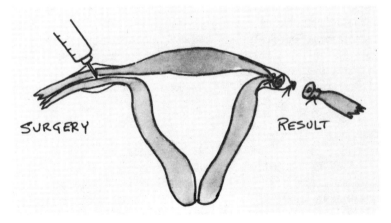

Figure 2-8   The Uchida resection

15

the distal stump is left projecting free into the peritoneal cavity. This complex procedure, although claimed to be 100% failure-free, has not become popular in the United States (Figure 2-8).

Fulguration

Although originally proposed as a method of tubal occlusion in 1937, electrodessication of a segment of tube has only come into common use in the past twenty years with the development of the modern fiberoptic laparoscope.[17,18] Using unipolar or bipolar grasping instruments, a high-frequency electric current (or, less often, thermocautery) is applied to the tube. This current produces permanent destruction of several centimeters of the tube and, if blended with a cutting current, can also divide the oviduct. Great care must be taken by the operator to avoid inadvertent burning of adjacent bowel or other organs by using only approved equipment (eg, electronic generators, noninsulating cannulas). For this procedure, the operator must possess a high level of technical training and skill.

Clipping

Suitable for all avenues of approach, the application of spring-loaded clips entails a low level of morbidity. Early models were associated with a high failure rate, probably caused by the then-available tantalum clips cutting through the tube and migrating away from the application site and by spontaneous spring failure.[19] Substitution of plastic clips closed by stainless steel springs[20] has increased the efficacy of this method; however, many otherwise skilled operators continue to find correct placement difficult (Figure 2-9).

Banding

This method, likewise suited for all approaches, involves the application of a small, tight, surgically inert, elastic band to a loop of fallopian tube. With a specialized applicator[21] a portion of the midsection of the tube is grasped and drawn into the surrounding sleeve; the elastic ring is then pushed over and onto the base of the

16

loop, thereby permanently occluding the lumen. Great skill is required to avoid lacerating the mesosalpinx and to assure a firm, tight fit well over the knuckle of the tube. Results are generally good with few failures or complications other than tubal transsection and immediate postoperative pain (probably secondary to anoxia of the occluded segment of tube) (Figure 2-10).

For our program, as described in this monograph, colpoceliotomy tubal sterilization utilizing a modification of the Kroener fimbriectomy was chosen as the best method, taking into account all of the advantages of the above-outlined procedures.

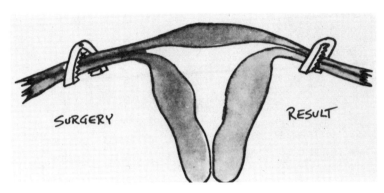

Figure 2-9   The clipping method

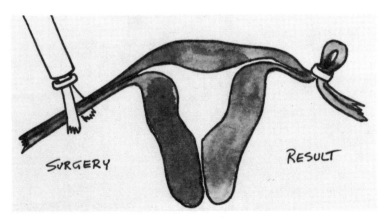

Figure 2-10   The banding method

Table 2-3
Comparison of Outpatient Surgical Sterilization Procedures[22]

Criteria	Laparoscopy (open or closed)	Mini-laparotomy	VTS
Equipment cost (1979)	$7500	$400	$400
Equipment maintenance	Complex	Simple	Simple
Skills required	Surgical with special training	Standard gyn training	Standard gyn training
Facility	Surgical center or operating room	Surgical center or operating room	Surgical center or operating room
Operative positioning	Semidorsal lithotomy & steep Trendelenburg	Semidorsal lithotomy or "frog-leg"	Standard dorsal lithotomy
Operating time	15-30 minutes	15-30 minutes	15-30 minutes

Anesthesia	General, spinal, local	General, spinal, local	General, spinal
Tubal closure technique	Electrocoagulation, Silastic band, clip	Segmental or fimbrial resection, Silastic band, clip	Segmental or fimbrial resection, Silastic band, clip
Recovery time (in facility)	1-6 hours	1-6 hours	1-6 hours
Skin scar	Yes	Yes	No
Tissue available for pathologic verification	No	Yes	Yes
Major complications	Uterine perforation, visceral burns, cardiac arrhythmia, visceral trauma (less with open)	Uterine perforation, bladder injury, visceral trauma, incisional hematoma and/or infection	Uterine perforation, vaginal hemorrhage

Mini-laparotomy remained the backup method of choice because, if the tubes cannot be reached from below or posteriorly, then they must be reached from above and anteriorly. Laparoscopy was performed only for those patients requesting this technique. The final choice of which method to use was based on preoperative evaluation, patient selection, occasionally on intraoperative circumstances, and on physician bias.

BIASES DEVELOPED IN THE COURSE OF EVALUATING OUR STERILIZATION PROGRAM

Certain personal biases developed in the course of evaluating this program. These might influence the choice of management of the surgical procedure.

Perhaps the most frequently cited reasons for the underutilization of the vaginal route for permanent contraception are the assertions that the vaginal approach is too difficult and that it entails problems in finding the oviducts, subsequently inducing the surgeon to use the abdominal route. A similar view had inhibited gynecologists from performing vaginal hysterectomy; yet once proven to be expeditious, technically not difficult, and well accepted by the patient, this technique became highly acceptable. VTS should likewise be accepted as a favored method for achievement of permanent contraception. Once it is taught as an accepted method, physicians will no longer fear or reject this most useful approach to the pelvic cavity and its contents.

Tubal sterilization should be a *nonreversible,* permanent procedure. The current effort to make tubal sterilization a reversible procedure is to be deplored. There appears to be a growing desire to live in a totally risk-free environment devoid of adverse consequences and guaranteed to give only favorable results. Total commitment or dedication to any decision seems to be out of date, and the proverbial back door through which one might wish to escape is sought by many. A choice of efficient methods of reversible contraception is already available to the well-motivated but undecided. "Minimal" segmental resection or occlusion, designed to permit subsequent reanastomosis, exposes the patient to greater hazards of primary surgical failure,[22] to the risks of yet another operation at great expense, as well as to the increased dangers of subsequent ectopic pregnancy (R.M. Lackritz, Assistant Clinical Professor of Obstetrics and Gynecology, U.T.H.S.C., San Antonio, Texas, personal communication, May 1980). Reconstructive tubal surgery should be reserved for those women made sterile from endometriosis, infection, or other inflammatory tubal damage (Table 2-3).

The presence of a surgical assistant is *mandatory*, regardless of the method of sterilization chosen. Unfortunately, the recent demand for cost-cutting has frequently led to the elimination of this assistant. This dangerous shortcut in the name of economy places the burden on the surgeon alone to perform surgery while struggling for exposure, thus prolonging operating time and placing the patient at greater risk from hemorrhage. We consider this to be medically unsound and foolish economy.

With the team approach we soon found that, after the entire team (surgeons, nurses, and anesthesiologist) had gained experience, we were able to complete each procedure in 10 to 15 minutes of actual operating time (25 to 30 minutes total time). Close communication between surgeons and anesthesiologist assured that the patient was sufficiently awake at the conclusion of the procedure to be extubated and to move herself from the operating table to the transport cart. This made day surgery safe and realistic with this procedure.

REFERENCES

1. Association for Voluntary Sterilization news release, New York, July 1979.
2. Rioux JE: Comment at Centennial Conference on Female Sterilization, Monterey, California, June 12, 1980.
3. Hassan HM: Open laparoscopy, in Phillips JM (ed). *Laparoscopy.* Baltimore, Williams and Wilkins, 1977.
4. Penfield AJ: *Female Sterilization by Mini-Laparotomy or Open Laparoscopy.* Baltimore, Urban and Schwartzenberg, 1980.
5. Center for Disease Control Surgical Surveillance Summary 1970–75, Atlanta, July 1979, p 7.
6. Miesfeld RR, Garratano RC, Moyers TG: Vaginal tubal ligation–is infection a significant risk? *Am J Obstet Gynecol* 137:183, 1980.
7. Wortman J: Tubal sterilization–review of methods. Population Reports, Washington University, Series C #7, May 1976, p c-76.

8. Lungren SS: A case of cesarean section twice successfully performed on the same patient, with remarks on the time, indications and details of the operation. *Am J Obstet Gynecol* 14:78, 1881.

9. Madlener M: Über sterilizierende Operazionen an den Tuben. *Zentralb Gynäk,* 43:380, 1919.

10. Stoot JEGM, Eubachs JMH: Sterilization by salpingectomy through posterior colpotomy. *Contraception* 8:577, 1973.

11. Bishop E, Nelms WF: A simple method of tubal sterilization, *NY State J Med* 39:214, 1930.

12. Garb AE: A review of tubal sterilization failure. *Obstet Gynecol Surv* 12:291, 1957.

13. Poulson AM: Analysis of female sterilization failure. *Obstet Gynecol* 42:131, 1973.

14. Kroener WF, Jr: Surgical sterilization by fimbriectomy, *Am J Obstet Gynecol* 104:247, 1969.

15. Irving FC: A new method of insuring sterility following Cesarean section. *Am J Obstet Gynecol* 8:335, 1924.

16. Uchida H: Uchida tubal sterilization. *Am J Obstet Gynecol* 121:153, 1975.

17. Rioux JE, Yutzpe AA: Electrosurgery untangled. *Contemp Obstet Gynecol* 4:118, 1974.

18. Ma HK, Wong V: Is occlusion of the fallopian tubes with tantalum clips a reversible and reliable method of sterilization? *Scott MJ* 19:183, 1974.

19. Hulka JF, et al: Sterilization by spring clip: A report of 1000 cases with a six month follow-up. *Fertil Steril* 26:1122, 1975.

20. Yoon IB, King TM: The laparoscopic Falope ring technique. *Adv Plann Parent* 10:154, 1975.

21. Stock JR: Tubal patency following Uchida tubal ligation: A histopathologic study of three cases. Presented at Armed Forces District-American College of Obstetricians and Gynecologists, October 3, 1979.

22. Lubell I, Frischer MS: Does mini-laparotomy for sterilization have a place in your practice? *Contemp Obstet Gynecol* 14:39, 1979.

3   History of Colpotomy Approach to Tubal Sterilization

Colpotomy, the incision in the anterior or posterior vaginal vault with the specific intent of entering the peritoneal cavity (colpoceliotomy), dates back to the nineteenth century. In their review Berger and Keith[1] make the point that culdotomy is a more accurate term for incision through the posterior vaginal fornix into the peritoneal cul-de-sac; however, most authors[2-9] writing about the vaginal route to female sterilization have settled on the posterior fornix approach and generally refer to this operation as colpotomy or colpoceliotomy. In 1831 the French gynecologist, Dr. Alfred J. Recamier,[10] used this approach to drain pelvic abscesses quite successfully. Dr. Ernst Wertheim,[11] a prominent Viennese gynecologist, performed many major gynecologic pelvic operations via the vaginal route toward the latter part of the nineteenth century. Another Viennese gynecologist, Friedrich Schauta[12] (to this day famous for his radical cancer surgery performed through the vagina), was active at about the same time. Toward the end of the nineteenth century (1895), Dr. Alfred Duhrssen,[13] a German surgeon, described a sexual tubal sterilization operation through the posterior colpotomy route. Interest waned until gynecology in the United States became a unique and separate discipline in the early years of the twentieth century. Population growth pressures, especially in India, prompted Asian physicians, notably Shirodkar, Soonawallah, and Purandare,[14] to reconsider the posterior colpotomy approach for tubal sterilization. Cross-fertilization of scientific minds during and after World War II stimulated experimentation in the United States with these allegedly "new and exotic" methods. Many reports (see text) of colpoceliotomy tubal sterilization have now appeared in the American medical literature.[1,15,16]

REFERENCES

1. Berger GS, Keith L: Culdotomy for female sterilization, *International Surgery* 62 (2) 72, 1977.
2. Ibid.
3. Brown HP, Schanzer SN: Vaginal tubal sterilization-lessons learned after 400 cases. Presented at Armed Forces District-American College of Obstetricians and Gynecologists, 18th Annual Meeting, October 1, 1979.
4. Hughes G, Liston WS: Comparison between laparoscopic sterilization and tubal ligation. *Br Med J* 2:637, 1975.
5. Kroener WF, Jr: Surgical sterilization by fimbriectomy. *Am J Obstet Gynecol* 112:247, 1969.
6. Metz KGP: Failures following fimbriectomy. *Fertil Steril* 28:66, 1977.
7. Metz KGP, Mastroianni L: Tubal pregnancy subsequent to transperitoneal migration of spermatozoa. *Obstet Gynecol Surv [Suppl]* 34:554, 1979.
8. Shepard MK: Female contraceptive sterilization. *Obstet Gynecol Surv* 29:739, 1974.
9. Wolf GC, Thompson NJ: Female sterilization and subsequent ectopic pregnancy. *Obstet Gynecol* 55:17, 1980.
10. Racamier, Alfred JCA, MD, France, 1774–1852, Gynecologist.
11. Wertheim, Ernst MD, Austria, 1864–1920, Gynecologist.
12. Schauta, Friedrich MD, Austria, 1849–1919, Gynecologist.
13. Duhrssen, Alfred MD, Germany, 1862–1933, Gynecologist.
14. Purandare VN: Evaluation of operative methods for female sterilization, presented at Conference on Family Planning and Biology of Reproduction, Bombay, India. March 3–8, 1969.

15. Shepard MK: Female contraceptive sterilization. *Obstet Gynecol Surv* 29:739, 1974.

16. Miesfeld RR, Garratano RC, Moyers TG: Vaginal tubal ligation. Is infection a significant risk? *Am J Obstet Gynecol* 137:183, 1980.

4   Alternatives to Vaginal Tubal Sterilization

CLOSED LAPAROSCOPY

Chronology

Laparoscopy for sterilization has been described and commonly practiced only in the past decade. In 1901 Kelling[1] first used the laparoscope as a diagnostic tool for examining the peritoneal cavity and viscera of dogs. In 1910 Jacobeus used the procedure on humans, coining the term "laparoscopy."[2] In 1930 Ruddock,[3] an American internist, became the main proponent of the procedure for diagnostic purposes. In 1937 Anderson[4] performed coagulation laparoscopic sterilization using endothermic coagulation.

Widespread clinical use was delayed until 1944 when Palmer[5] introduced intrauterine probes and biopsy forceps and stressed intraabdominal pressure monitoring. However, not until the development of fiberoptic, cold light sources in the late 1960s did laparoscopic sterilization by fulguration become popular in the United States.

Operative Technique

After a skin and vaginal prep, the patient is placed in the Trendelenburg and modified dorsal lithotomy position. Bimanual pelvic exam is performed, a uterine manipulator (Hulka, Sargis, or similar) placed, and the bladder catheterized; the catheter is left in place. After making an incision in the lower portion of the umbilicus (through fascia), a Verres (or similar needle is used to establish pneumoperitoneum with either carbon dioxide or nitrous oxide gas. After satisfactory insufflation to achieve abdominal wall elevation, a metal-sleeved, sharp-pointed trocar is introduced into the peritoneal cavity. This intraabdominal placement is accomplished with a controlled thrust, following which a telescope is inserted to allow panoramic inspection of the pelvis. The fallopian tubes are then grasped with an appropriate instrument through either an operating channel or a second smaller puncture (made in the lower abdomen under visual guidance). For tubal closure, the operator has the choice of unipolar or bipolar coagulation, banding with elastic rubber rings, or clip application (modified Hulka or similar). Once satisfactory tubal occlusion and hemostasis have been established, the cannula(s) is withdrawn, evacuating as much gas as possible. The incision(s) is closed with subcutaneous sutures and either subcuticular closure or skin clips. The incision(s) is usually coverable with Band-Aids, hence the common name for this type of surgery.

Anesthesia

General endotracheal or local field block (the latter requiring the use of less gas but mandating bands or clips) is used. General anesthesia by mask is contraindicated because of gastric distention and possible hypercapnia leading to cardiac arrhythmia.

Contraindications for closed laparoscopy include marked obesity; a history of multiple abdominal surgery or generalized peritonitis; umbilical, abdominal, or diaphragmatic hernias; and cardiovascular and/or respiratory disease.

One of the attested advantages is that an assistant is not required, although we firmly disagree with this for reasons discussed elsewhere. Operating time is brief and postoperative recovery is rapid, making this method suitable for outpatient day surgery in a hospital or surgical center. We do not believe doctors' offices or free-standing clinics are safe places for this procedure.[5,6] An important advantage is the usefulness of the laparoscope for diagnostic purposes; the view it provides is rivaled only by open laparotomy.

The major disadvantages of closed laparoscopy are that it is a blind approach to entering the abdominal cavity and entails the concomitant risk to intraperitoneal structures including bowel and blood vessels. The equipment used is expensive, complex, and difficult to maintain in perfect working order. The use of intraperitoneal gas, together with the steep Trendelenburg position needed for clear viewing of the pelvis, creates anesthetic hazards of cardiac arrhythmia and difficult ventilation. This method also requires a high degree of surgical skill acquired only after an extensive and supervised training period.

Complications occur in about 1% to 2% of cases. They may be early or late. The early complications are due to lacerations of the cervix or perforations of the uterus by the cervical manipulator, or to a failure to achieve intraabdominal pneumoperitoneum; the ensuing subcutaneous emphysema could lead to cardiac arrhythmias from hypercapnia. The blindly inserted trocar can cause blood vessel or bowel lacerations. Other intraabdominal injuries can be caused by direct burns to adjacent loops of bowel or to more distant organs such as the bladder by "creeping" high-frequency electric currents (0.2% to 1.3% of cases using high-frequency fulguration[7]). The wrong structures (eg, the round ligament) can be transsected, resulting in brisk intraperitoneal bleeding. Postoperative pain from peritoneal irritation or traction is not uncommon.

The late complications of the procedure include torsion of the distal end of the fallopian tube, bilateral hydrosalpinx, intrauterine or extrauterine pregnancy (intrauterine in 1 out of 2,000 cases[8] or extrauterine in up to 90% of failures[9]), a vague and ill-defined alteration in the menstrual flow (the post-tubal-ligation syndrome, see Chapter 11, Long-term follow-up), and umbilical hernia formation.

OPEN LAPAROSCOPY

First described in 1977, this procedure is a modification of the closed laparoscopy technique and developed to its present state of the art by Hassan.[10] The surgical procedure utilizes a small incision, under direct vision, through the infraumbilical fascia to allow advancing the cannula and laparoscope into the peritoneum under direct visual control. Pneumoperitoneum is introduced only after the cannulas and telescope are in place, thus avoiding blind stabs into the abdomen with either sharp trocar or needle. The management of the tubes is the same as with closed laparoscopy.

Contraindications are the same as with closed laparoscopy, although this may be possible in individuals with a history of multiple abdominal operations and/or adhesions. The failure rate is the same as in open laparoscopy.

The advantages of open laparoscopy are: the insertion of the cannula and laparoscope is safe, layered closures ensure the prevention of postoperative herniation, and the procedure may be suitable to free-standing clinics or the physician's office.[6] Once entry into the peritoneal cavity has been achieved, visualization through the telescope is identical with that in closed laparoscopy.

The disadvantage of this procedure is that it requires an assistant (in our view an advantage). Except for the insertion, the procedure is similar to closed laparoscopy.

The complications are the same as for closed laparoscopy except that with the open technique trocar injuries are avoided and pneumoperitoneum is more readily achieved.

MINI-LAPAROTOMY

Chronology

Although originally described by Blundell in the early nineteenth century,[11] the first modern description was made by Uchida in 1971.[12] The American adaptation of the technique, using general anesthesia, was first described by Saunders and Munsick in 1972.[13] In 1973 Osathanonda pioneered the mini-laparotomy under local anesthesia and in free-standing clinics.[14]

Operative Technique

The patient is placed in either the "frog-leg" or semi-lithotomy position. The bladder is catheterized and the catheter is left in place. An intrauterine manipulator (Vitoon, Hulka, Sargis, or similar) is placed and elevated to palpate the uterine fundus through the abdominal wall. (If the fundus is not palpable the procedure will be difficult if not impossible.)[6] A 3-cm incision is made in the suprapubic skin fold. The uterus is elevated to the incision and rotated to expose the tubes in turn. The tubes are hooked digitally or by instrument and elevated with Babcock clamps. Tubal closure is most frequently accomplished by the Pomeroy technique, but elastic rubber banding, placement of clips, or fimbriectomy are also applicable. The incision is closed in layers with catgut or polyglycolate sutures. An assistant is mandatory.

Contraindications to mini-laparotomy are gross obesity, fixed uterine retroversion secondary to either endometriosis or chronic pelvic inflammation, leiomyomata uteri, or other pelvic or large adnexal disease.

Advantages include the simplicity of this easy-to-learn technique, the use of standard instrumentation (with the exception of the intrauterine manipulator), minimal maintenance requirements, and a high degree of safety for the patient which makes possible the use of surgical facilities in doctors' offices or free-standing clinics. There are few disadvantages. The tubes are not always easily found, requiring considerable searching with resultant tubal trauma; this is especially true in the obese female.

31

Complications include uterine perforation with the manipulator, the previously mentioned tubal and mesosalpingeal injuries, bladder lacerations, and even occasionally bowel injury. With the use of local anesthesia, vasovagal syncope has been reported.

VAGINAL HYSTERECTOMY: A VIABLE INPATIENT ALTERNATIVE TO TUBAL STERILIZATION

Chronology and Technique

The development and the surgical techniques are well described in standard textbooks of operative gynecology and are beyond the scope of this monograph. We maintain that there is a legitimate place for vaginal hysterectomy for voluntary sterilization. Usually the patient requesting permanent sterilization is a multipara with concomitant vaginal or rectal wall relaxation or descensus uteri or other clinical or anatomic uterine pathology (eg, menometrorrhagia from ovarian dysfunction, adenomyosis, or leiomyomata. At this time in life cancer fears become more real and conception is considered totally unacceptable. Under these circumstances, vaginal hysterectomy with or without added colpoperineoplasty definitely has its place.

As with vaginal hysterectomy for other reasons, contraindications include excessive uterine size either from fibroids or adenomyosis, fixed retroversion either from endometriosis or chronic inflammation, or high fixation of the uterus from surgical or other causation.[15]

The advantages of this approach include the almost complete absence of any postoperative failures (pregnancy), although tubal and even abdominal pregnancies occasionally occur. The concomitant correction of abnormal anatomic conditions and total avoidance of future cervical or endometrial cancer make this approach very attractive in selected patients. The disadvantages of this method, in comparison with tubal sterilization, lie in an increased morbidity and mortality, the necessity of in-hospital stay, prolonged recovery time, the added expense, and the prohibition of federal funding for voluntary sterilization by hysterectomy.

ALTERNATE, REVERSIBLE, AND OTHER METHODS OF CONCEPTION CONTROL

Oral Contraceptives

Oral synthetic estrogenic and progestogenic hormone combinations presently are the most effective reversible methods of preventing unwanted pregnancy (less than 1% theoretical failure but use-failure rate of 4%).[16] In addition, they very effectively control excessive, painful, and irregular menses. This method of birth control is not dependent on the patient's usage immediately prior to intercourse. Complications are rare but can be serious (eg, thromboembolism and vascular accidents). The pill should probably not be used by women over 35, especially if they are tobacco smokers.[17] Women with strong family histories of diabetes, coronary disease, or hypertension are also at a greater risk for vascular complications.

Intrauterine Devices (IUD)

These are very effective devices which are placed in the uterine cavity. There are two types: nonmedicated which can be left in utero for an indefinite length of time; and medicated (eg, progesterone-releasing or copper-wrapped which have a one-to-three-years effective time). They offer 97% to 99% protection against unwanted pregnancy[18] although an increase in tubal pregnancies has been reported. A further advantage is that they are maintenance free. The primary disadvantages are development of occasionally serious pelvic infections and possible spontaneous expulsion or transmigration of the device. The medicated IUDs must be replaced periodically to maintain effectiveness.

Other Methods

Injections of long-acting progestational hormone (primarily medroxyprogesterone acetate) every three months is highly protective and very cost-effective. Unfortunately, it is not yet authorized by the US Food and Drug Administration in spite of its high patient acceptability, extreme efficiency, and use in family planning programs in 82 other countries.[19]

Intrauterine application of sclerosing agents such as quinacrine hydrochloride, intratubal injection of thermosetting plastics, and cyanomethacrylate plugs has been used. All of these are at present experimental, but with increasingly sophisticated hysteroscopes they may well become the ideal reversible methods of the future.[20]

POSTPARTUM STERILIZATION

Postpartum Tubal Sterilization

Permanent tubal sterilization can readily be performed at the time of cesarean section or in the 12 to 24 hours after vaginal delivery. There are obvious reasons for doing the surgical procedure at this time: (1) The patient is already hospitalized for the obstetrical delivery. (2) An additional day adds little to the cost of hospitalization. (No additional postoperative stay is required after cesarean section.) With day-care surgery in Surgi-Centers available to cut costs, this is no longer as important as it was before outpatient sterilization became popular. (3) The request for puerperal sterilization logically follows the patient's decision made either prior to conception or during pregnancy that she now has completed her family and wishes no future pregnancies. (4) Few, if any, postoperative restrictions need be added to the usual postpartum limitations. (5) Morbidity and mortality from immediate postdelivery tubal sterilization is negligible.

However, sterilization immediately following delivery may in some cases be very ill-timed. The patient may be motivated by emotional rather than intellectual factors under pressure from the obstetrical experience, especially if the pregnancy was difficult or uncomfortable. A high rate of regret and request for reversal of tubal sterilization in this category of patients attests to this fact.[6] Tubal sterilizations performed at the time of cesarean section and in the immediate postpartum period reportedly have a higher failure rate than interval procedures. The reasons for this are unclear but may be related to the succulent state of tissues at that time with subsequent shrinkage and loosening of suture ties. Infant mortality is highest in the first 28 days of life. An irreversible procedure blocking fertility performed immediately after birth does not allow the mother the flexibility of action necessary after such an untoward event.

The procedure is performed similarly to any tubal sterilization done via standard or mini-laparotomy, although certain authors advocate the use of the laparoscope even at this time.[21,22] Obviously, the grossly enlarged postpartum uterus and the succulent and friable state of the vaginal and parametrial tissues make the colpotomy approach impossible.

Technique for Tubal Ligation at the Time of Cesarean Section

After completion of the cesarean section and closure of the uterine incision, the fallopian tubes are exposed in turn, clamped, cut, and tied by the chosen tubal closure technique as with any other route of approach. Elastic bands or spring-loaded clips may also be satisfactory, provided the tubes are not too edematous. The existence of higher postpartum failure rates as discussed above must be taken into account.

Technique for Tubal Ligation After Vaginal Delivery

Entry into the peritoneal cavity is made either via a short, vertical, midline, infraumbilical incision or via a semicircular, intraumbilical approach to its lower circumference, as appropriate. Any major anesthesia as well as local anesthesia (in selected patients) is acceptable; care must be taken to avoid injury to the bowel upon entry into the peritoneal cavity due to laxity and the splayed-out condition of the puerperal abdominal wall. Since the fallopian tubes are especially enlarged and succulent at this time, extra caution and gentleness in handling is required. The incision is closed in the usual manner with special attention to the reapproximation of the rectus sheath to avoid infraumbilical herniation. The skin may be closed with clips or a subcuticular suture.[22]

REFERENCES

1. Kelling A, in Horwitz ST: Laparoscopy in gynecology, *Obstet Gynecol Surv* 27:1, 1972.

2. Jacobeus A, in Aronson AR, Parker GW: Peritoneoscopy: Its value as a diagnostic aid. *Am J Dig Dis* 5:931, 1960.

3. Ruddock W, in Horwitz ST: Laparoscopy in gynecology, *Obstet Gynecol Surv* 27:1, 1972.

4. Anderson ET: Peritoneoscopy. *Am J Surg* 35:136, 1937.

5. Palmer R, in Marlow J: Laparoscopy. *Med Ann DC*, 41:162, 1972.

6. Penfield AJ: *Female Sterilization by Mini-Laparotomy or Open Laparoscopy.* Baltimore, Urban and Schwarzenberg, 1980.

7. Rioux JE, Yutzpe AA: Electrosurgery untangled. *Contemp Obstet Gynecol* 4:118, 1974.

8. McCausland A: Ectopic pregnancy following tubal ligation. *Am J Obstet Gynecol* 135:97, 1980.

9. Wolf GC, Thompson NJ: Female sterilization and subsequent ectopic pregnancy. *Obstet Gynecol* 55:17, 1980.

10. Hassan HM: Open laparoscopy; in Phillips JM (ed): *Laparoscopy,* Baltimore, Williams and Wilkins, 1977.

11. Blundell J, in Speert H: *Essays in Eponymy,* New York, Macmillan, 1958, p 620.

12. Uchida H: Uchida sterilization in family planning; in Hudodo ST, Saifadduin AB (eds): *Fifth Asian Congress of Obstetrics and Gynecology,* Djakarta, October 8, 1971, p 157–158.

13. Saunders WG, Munsick RA: Non-puerperal female sterilization. *Obstet Gynecol* 40:443, 1972.

14. Osathanonda V: Supra-pubic mini-laparotomy *Contraception* 10:251, 1974.

15. Gray LA: *Vaginal hysterectomy.* Second edition, Springfield, Ill., Charles C Thomas, 1963, p 71.

16. Ryder B: Contraceptive failure in the United States, *Fam Plann Perspect* 5:133, 1973.

17. Tietze C: New estimates of mortality associated with fertility control, *Fam Plann Persepct* 9:74, 1977.

18. Ryder Norman B: Contraceptive failure in the United States, *Fam Plann Perspect* 5:133, 1973.

19. Hatcher RA: *Contraceptive Technology 1980-81* New York, Irvington Publishers, Inc., 1980, p 45.

20. Wortman J: Tubal Sterilization–review of methods, Population Reports Series C #7, Washington, DC, US Government Printing Office, 1976, p c-81.

21. Keith L, Webster A, Houser K et al: Laparoscopy for puerperal sterilization, *Obstet Gynecol* 39:616, 1972.

22. Whitely PF: Laparoscopic sterilization in the puerperium *J Obstet Gynecol Br Commonwealth* 79:166, 1972.

5 Patient Preparation

PATIENT FLOW

The first contact with the patient is usually by telephone, although some patients will have made an on-site visit at the referral agency. At this time the request for voluntary sexual tubal sterilization is registered, and the patient is told when to return for her first counseling session. She is also given a very broad overview of the procedure, and financial entitlements are checked and categorized.

The first formal session shortly after the initial contact consists of group counseling by a trained counselor as well as audiovisual presentations (see Appendix 1) of tubal sterilizations. Complete entitlements (Federal Social Security Act Titles XIX and XX) or other third-party payers are evaluated and recorded. Blood is drawn for hemoglobin-hematocrit determination and for syphilis serologic testing. A chest roentgenogram is scheduled to be taken a few days preoperatively at the hospital where the tubal sterilization will be done. A permission for operation form is signed.

In order to comply with federal guidelines[1] of a 30-day "cooling off" period between counseling and operating, the next visit is not scheduled until three weeks later. At this time one of us (Dr. Brown or Dr. Schanzer) will see the patient and perform a thorough history evaluation and physical examination. He will also

Table 5-1
Patient Flow in a Sterilization Program

Visit	Activities	Time Intervals
Initial contact	Information (in person/phone) Individual counseling	
I	Group counseling (by counselor) Laboratory work: hematocrit serology chest roentgenogram Entitlements (Titles XIX & XX) Permission forms	
II	History and physical exam Laboratory work: Pap smear gonorrhea culture pregnancy test & review of previous lab data Group counseling (by physician)	30 days by federal regulation
		7 days
	Surgical Procedure	
		14 days
III	Follow-up visit: Interim history and physical exam Laboratory work: pregnancy test other tests (as indicated)	

review previously obtained laboratory results, obtain material from the uterine cervix for gonorrhea culture, Pap smear, and order a pregnancy test.[2] When all patients of this group have been seen, the physician will assemble them for a detailed group-counseling session. All counseling sessions with the patients must be completely documented. After a final week of preoperative waiting (to complete the 30-day delay) the patients arrive at the hospital for surgery. The period at the hospital will be covered in detail in later chapters.

Two weeks after the operation, the patients are again examined and questioned as to possible adverse reactions or results; this is done at the referral clinic and performed by a licensed nurse-practitioner. In the event of the discovery of significant abnormalities, the patient is so informed and referred back to the operating surgeon. Final laboratory work ordered at this last visit includes a pregnancy test and other such tests as might be indicated (hemoglobin-hematocrit, gonorrhea culture, other bacteriologic cultures, etc.).

A minimum of four visits are needed to complete the required components of this program. Prior to the institution of the federal 30-day delay regulation in 1979, the first two visits were combined, allowing for the then required 72-hour delay rule. These guidelines apply to federally subsidized programs and could easily be modified for application in the private sector of American medicine as well as in other countries of the world. Table 5-1 presents a summary of the above in flow-sheet form.

COUNSELING FOR STERILIZATION

Philosophy

Permanent prevention of fertility should be available to mature, competent women who have full knowledge of reversible methods of fertility control and an understanding of male sterilization. No patient should be refused sterilization solely because of age (except where services are paid by federal or Texas Title XX funds), nulliparity, race, marital status, or economic status. It should be noted that, as of this writing, no reference text exists on counseling for sterilization. Therefore, each facility needs to develop guidelines best suited to its clients' socioeconomic class and community.

Patient processing is initiated with individual counseling and later in groups by specially trained counselors who discuss the basics of reproductive physiology and anatomy, the choice of operations available, and other physical and emotional sequelae (or lack thereof) of tubal sterilization. Liberal use is made of audiovisual aids (see Appendix 1). Spouses or partners are encouraged to accompany the patient at the counseling session.

After a complete history and physical examination performed by the operating surgeon, another group-counseling session with the physician is held, where informed consent is obtained. Records of such sessions must be documented by counselors and physicians.

The following are pertinent points for physician discussion with the patients.

1. The physician explains the physiology of conception and how tubal occlusion prevents conception while preserving menstrual and sexual function.
2. The three main approaches to the fallopian tubes (laparoscopy, mini-laparotomy, and vaginal approach) are explained and medical reasons are given why specific routes are chosen.
3. The complications to be expected with the various approaches and a statement of the surgeon's biases are set forth.
4. There is a frank discussion of failure (pregnancy), including the options of obstetric delivery, subsequent termination, and reoperation.
5. If tubal sterilization is rejected, alternate operations (hysterectomy, pregnancy termination) versus available medical techniques of contraception are discussed.
6. Male sterilization is presented as a viable alternative to tubal sterilization.
7. Previous contraceptive experiences and failures are discussed and the patient is asked how she arrived at her decision for permanent contraception.

8. The irreversible nature of the procedure is indicated.
9. The impact of the sterilization on future marriages, changes in partners, or death of an existent child is considered.
10. Patients are given an opportunity to ask questions as well as the option to change their minds at any time prior to surgery.
11. Preoperative patient instruction is provided (see Chapter 8).

Male Versus Female Sterilization

Where no pathology exists in either partner and both are willing to accept sterilization, there is ample justification for recommending that the male partner be sterilized for the following reasons:

1. The vasectomy procedure is at least as effective in the prevention of pregnancy as is tubal ligation.
2. Vasectomy is a rapid, simple, subcutaneous surgical procedure almost always suited to local anesthesia, whereas tubal ligation involves the invasion of one of the body's deepest recesses and, under most circumstances, is not suitable to local anesthesia.
3. Men who are willing and comfortable in the knowledge that they will experience no change in sexual function, attitude, or general health rarely regret having the procedure done.
4. In spite of multiple investigations[3] over the past fifty years as to whether health would be threatened in one way or another as a result of vasectomy, as of this writing no substantiated data exist that any specific disease process is caused or enhanced by vasectomy.

If, in the evaluation of the patient, it becomes apparent that she is not dedicated to the idea of permanent contraception, she should be rejected as a candidate for surgery. Situations leading to ambiguity include chronological or emotional immaturity, recent pregnancy, peer or spouse pressure, financial distress, recent widowhood or abandonment, and the lack of commitment to a final decision. Allowing an undecided patient to become permanently sterilized can only lead to regret at a future date or possible legal involvement of the surgeon.

At no time should a patient be coerced into accepting tubal sterilization. She must be allowed to form her own decision based on all available considerations and should be given the opportunity to return at a future date for reconsideration or be referred for counseling. Of course, appropriate contraceptive advice must be given before dismissal from the program.

QUESTIONS AND ANSWERS DURING COUNSELING OF VTS PATIENTS

The following are actual questions which have been raised during preoperative group counseling sessions:

Question   Am I sterile immediately after surgery? If so, why do I have to wait two weeks before having intercourse?

Answer   Sterility is achieved immediately by surgery; therefore, no other birth control should ever be necessary. The recommended delay in resuming intercourse is to insure complete healing of the internal and/or external incisions; they could be injured during intercourse, leading to hemorrhage or infection.

Question   Will my periods be changed by the operation?

Answer   Under usual circumstances, no. A small percentage of women with tubal ligations (by any of the usual methods) have been reported to develop menstrual abnormalities. At present, researchers have been unable to establish a definite relationship between tubal surgery and menstrual periods. Scant vaginal bleeding can be expected for two to ten days postoperatively. The age of onset of menopause is not changed.

Question   Will I have severe pain or feel sick after the operation?

Answer   Mild to moderate pain, such as cramps, aching in the pelvis, and premenstrual-like pressure, is frequently experienced for 24 to 48 hours. Almost always the pain is relieved by mild analgesics such as acetaminophen. Avoid aspirin in the immediate postoperative period; it alters your blood's ability to clot and therefore may make you bleed more than necessary. If the pain is persistent or severe in spite of mild analgesics, you should notify your surgeon or clinic since this is an unusual and possibly important development. A "washed-out" feeling is usual in many patients for 24 to 48 hours after surgery; a mild, scratchy, sore throat may be present for about 24 hours.

Question Other than avoiding intercourse, are there any other activities I can or cannot do after surgery?

Answer In general, strenuous activities should be avoided for 24 to 48 hours postoperatively. Most patients return to their usual work comfortably within 48 hours. Tub baths or showers may be taken at any time.

Question Why is a postoperative exam necessary?

Answer An examination two weeks postoperatively is necessary to confirm satisfactory incisional healing and absence of vaginal infection, and to discuss any operative findings which need clarification for future preventive health maintenance. You should continue to make an annual visit to your physician or clinic for an exam and Pap smear.

Question Will I feel different after my surgery?

Answer In the vast majority of cases, women report themselves unchanged physically and psychologically. A few report a sense of relief and greater freedom of sexual expression. Some women will have short-term feelings of uneasiness at having taken this permanent step. Those women who continue to feel regretful after surgery are usually the ones who felt that way before or had the operation as a result of familial, financial, or social pressures. It is this group of women for whom a delay period between counseling and the actual operation has been set aside. Yet, in spite of careful evaluation and counseling, 1% of the women who had tubal sterilization subsequently request that tubal "untying" be performed.

Question If infection is a possible complication, what are the signs?

Answer   Pelvic infection causes many of the classical signs found in infections elsewhere in the body, ie, fever (temperature greater than 100° F by mouth), generalized aching, pelvic pain, a yellow vaginal discharge. A bloody or yellow discharge can occur even in the absence of infection when the vaginal suture line heals unusually slowly or "granulates." This latter condition may be annoying but is not dangerous and is easily treated in the office or clinic. Pelvic infection, however, is potentially serious yet responds rapidly to antibiotics if treatment is started early.

Question   Should I worry if my period comes early?

Answer   Tubal sterilization alone does not usually alter the interval between periods. Occasionally the vaginal suture line begins to bleed about 12 to 14 days after surgery. Usually this is easily controlled in the office or clinic with little or no pain for the patient.

Question   Will I lose my "nature" by this operation?

Answer   No, sex drive is unaffected by this surgery, as are sensations or enjoyment during intercourse. Possibly there may be an improvement, knowing that you are safe from pregnancy.

Question   Can my tubes be "untied"?

Answer   Theoretically, yes. However, the surgery involved to restore tubes to the open state is complicated, prolonged, expensive, and only about 50% effective. In those conceiving, 5% to 10% of the pregnancies may be tubal rather than uterine in implantation, creating a major threat to the woman's life. Therefore, it is best to have clearly and definitively made up one's mind before surgery, rather than have subsequent regrets and request for untying the tubes.

Question   Will I still have menstrual periods after the operation?

Answer   The operation for tying the tubes closes the fallopian tubes mechanically, thereby preventing the union of the sperm and egg; it in no way alters the cyclic hormonal release from the pituitary gland and ovaries, the events which result in the monthly bleeding.

Question   If I am on the pill before surgery, when will I have to stop taking it?

Answer   If your pill contains less than 80 μg of estrogen, do not stop the pill before surgery but continue to finish the cycle. Just do not start a new package. If you are on one of the strong pills (more than 80 μg), these should be stopped for a month before surgery, and other effective methods of contraception such as foam and condoms should be used.

Question   If I have an IUD, what do I have to do?

Answer   The IUD should be removed at least one month before the surgery date to allow for at least one normal menstrual period to occur. Of course, you must prevent an interval pregnancy by using foam and condoms in combination.

Question   Will this operation make me gain weight?

Answer   Only if you begin to eat more than before your operation.

Question   What will happen to the egg if the tubes are blocked?

Answer   The egg, as important to reproduction as it is, is a tiny structure about the size of a pin head. It falls into the abdominal cavity, dissolves, and is eventually reabsorbed. An estimated 20% to 30% of eggs fall into the abdominal cavity with open tubes.

Question   Can a woman who has never had children have a tubal sterilization?

Answer   There are no laws in any state prohibiting voluntary sterilization for mentally competent, consenting adults. Many physicians and clinics are reluctant to sterilize women who have never borne children (as they are to sterilize women under 29 or recently separated) as these women have been shown to be likely to change their minds after surgery or feel regretful and ask for untying of their tubes.

Question   How come the operation cannot be guaranteed to prevent pregnancy?

Answer   One to five women out of 1000 having had tubal sterilization may become pregnant. Most of them conceive by the first postoperative year, but some may get pregnant as long as five years later. In spite of the best screening, some women may already be pregnant at the time of surgery. Upon investigation, the cause of the opening between the tube and the abdominal cavity is frequently not identifiable. The only surgery that can guarantee sterility is a hysterectomy, a longer, more complicated, and more expensive operation. (The federal government refuses to pay for hysterectomy solely for the purpose of sterilization.)

REFERENCES

1. Department of Health Education and Welfare, Fiscal Division, Federal Sterilization Regulations, 42 CFR, part 441, subsection F, February, 1979.

2. Pregnosis, Roche Diagnostics, Hoffmann–LaRoche, Nutley, New Jersey.

3. Davis J, Jr: Centennial Conference on Female Sterilization in the U.S.A., Monterey, California, June 1980.

6 Medical-Legal Considerations in Tubal Sterilization

GENERAL CONSIDERATIONS

In an attempt to minimize litigational complications following sexual sterilization, hospitals and physicians have established certain criteria or safeguards consisting of restraints imposed by committees and government regulations; on the whole these are designed to asssure quality medical care, safeguard patient interests, and, or course, reduce legal involvement.

Sterilization may be divided into four major categories: punitive, eugenic, therapeutic, and contraceptive.

Punitive Sterilization

Although this form of sterilization has been used in times past, recent awareness of personal liberties and rights has stopped this practice.

Eugenic Sterilization

There is a wide divergence of legal opinion regarding sterilization for eugenic reasons. Ideally, if one could prevent propagation of undesirable genetic traits by forced sterilization, then a nation consisting of a "pure, untainted super race" could gradually evolve. Where is one to draw the line? Mental defectives with obvious chromosomal abnormalities? Imbeciles with low I.Q.? Diabetics? Shades of Nazi Germany cloud this issue. Yet some states still adhere to Justice Holmes's opinion that "three generations of imbeciles are enough", and permit limited eugenic sterilizations.[1]

The sexual sterilization of the mentally retarded and minors for eugenic purposes in the United States remains an unresolved issue ethically; legally it is prohibited.[2] Under circumstances of "liberation" (independent maintenance, marriage, etc.), voluntary sterilization may be legally and ethically defensible for minors in cases where government funds are not requested. When a mentally-retarded female is unable to care for herself during menstruation, a hysterectomy can often be justified and, of course, provides the added protection from unwanted pregnancy. Great care must be used, however, in recommending this approach.

Therapeutic Sterilization

Such sterilizations are performed for "medical necessity," eg, progressive diabetes mellitus or multiple sclerosis. Since medical necessity is hard to define clearly and since the criteria are becoming more stringent, a physician would do well to consider this kind of surgical procedure most carefully lest he or she be accused of malpractice at a future date.

Contraceptive Failure

Except in the case of the retarded and minors (under 18 or in some states, 21 years of age), there are no state laws prohibiting voluntary sexual sterilizations; there are no mandatory 30-day delay regulations for nonfederally funded sterilizations. The recent federal regulations[1] decree that sterilizations cannot be performed sooner than 30 days or later than 180 days from the date of consent except in cases of premature obstetric delivery or emergency abdominal surgery; prior regulations required only a 72-hour waiting period.[2] The avowed intent of these delay mandates is to allow the recipient of federal funds ample time to change her mind and prevent subsequent regret in having made the wrong decision. During the initial 19 months of our program, we functioned under the 72-hour rule. Our estimate of the patient change-of-mind rate for that period was 7% (our entire drop-out rate for that period). During the subsequent 11 months under the new 30-day delay period, the patient change-of-mind rate rose to 17%, but the overall drop-out rate rose to 33%. Since 16% of the initially processed patients never returned and could not be located, the actual number of patients who conceived because of this arbitrary ruling is unknown.

It is our impression that this legislation is counterproductive for the following reasons: (1) A second preoperative visit was needed to complete the arrangements in proper sequence; this additional visit was also necessary to ensure that the patient would not be pregnant at the time of surgery and was free of gonorrheal infection and cervical neoplasia. This contributed additional expense to the total cost of services. (2) Rather than inhibiting providers from coercing patients into overly hasty decisions, the new rule allows for the occurrence of unwanted pregnancies in a population which can least afford it. Not only does this add unnecessary costs to the tax and welfare burden all American citizens must bear; it also forces these unfortunate women to carry pregnancies to term, creating an end-result *completely opposite* to the originally desired intent.

A return to the 72-hour delay rule would continue to safeguard adequately against prematurely performed tubal ligations, yet still reduce the number of unwanted conceptions. Our views coincide with those of the Association of Planned Parenthood Physicians.[3]

Further requirements of these federal regulations are: (1) A consent form, clearly explaining the nature and consequences in a language the patient understands, approved by the Department of Health, Education and Welfare (now the Department of Health and Human Services), must be used. (2) Consent may not be obtained from anyone in labor of childbirth, under the influence of alcohol or other drugs, or seeking or obtaining an abortion. (3) Patients undergoing hysterectomy for any reason must be advised orally and in writing that sterility will result. Medicaid (Title XIX) payment will not be made for hysterectomy performed for the sole purpose of sterilizing the individual. (4) Special arrangements must be made for the handicapped individual. (5) Federal funding will not be available for sterilization of individuals institutionalized in correctional facilities, mental hospitals, or other rehabilitative facilities. (6) The prohibition against using federal funds to pay for the sterilization of individuals judged mentally incompetent by a court and those under 21 years of age is continued.

Many countries have no legal guidelines regarding sterilizations, allowing family planning programs to be effectively introduced. Other countries have legislative codes pertaining to surgical sterilizations, such as age requirements, restrictions on personnel performing these operations, and the facilities where they may be performed.

HUSBAND'S CONSENT

Although the spouse's consent is not legally mandated prior to voluntary sterilizations, most physicians and clinics attempt to obtain it to avoid animosity or threatened legal entanglement. For a summary of sterilization consent requirements see Table 6-1. For examples of private-sector and federally authorized consent forms, see Appendix 2.

CRIMINAL AND CIVIL LIABILITIES

Criminal Liability

There are no longer any states in the United States where sterilization procedures are against the law.[4] It is unlikely that a physician could be held liable in a sterilization operation if the patient has given full consent; doctrines "contrary to public policy or

Table 6-1
Sterilization Consent Requirements

Category	Legally Correct	Federal and/or State Funds Allowed	Remarks
Over 21, consenting, competent	yes	yes	...
Less than 21, competent	no	no	Possible under court order, but actually
Mentally retarded, dependent	no	no	impossible to obtain
Single	yes	yes	...
Separated	yes	yes	Spouse consent not required

national interest" would not likely be invoked by a public prosecutor. Likewise, an accusation of "assault or mayhem" could no longer be used against a physician if he or she is protected by a voluntarily signed document of permission.

Civil Liability

A physician can be held liable for untoward results of tubal sterilization if his standard of care falls below that of any prudent practitioner in the United States. Only damage resulting from this substandard action of failure to accomplish the contractually agreed-upon act is sufficient grounds for a civil tort suit.[5]

Presently there are eight unresolved cases of litigation[6] pertaining to unsuccessful sterilization attempts. Two main issues are involved: (1) the concept of "wrongful birth" (or wrongful conception or pregnancy), and (2) lack of clearly understood informed consent. In neither case is the issue one of surgical ineptness but rather one of failure to produce the desired end-result, namely permanent infertility. In other words, a *breach of contract* to sterilize the *plaintiff-mother* occurred. The existence of one's fundamental right to sue for such a breach of contract has been established. That a birth resulting from this unwanted and unplanned pregnancy constitutes a substantial interference with the fundamental right of the parents has been granted by the US Supreme Court which thus provides a legal remedy. Savage[6] feels that allowing recovery of the costs entailed in raising this healthy but unwanted child constitutes gross legal and moral malpractice, that not every wrong has an associated remedy, that placing legal blame on the physician simply means that he or she is a convenient "fall guy," and that this is not sufficient cause for a malpractice action.

The best defense against this kind of legal blackmail is a totally frank preoperative discussion of operative failures, complications, and hazards; its keystone must be a *fully informed consent.*

REFERENCES

1. Gambell RJ: Legal status of therapeutic abortion and sterilization in the US, *Clin Obstet Gynecol* 7:22, 1974.

2. Department of Health, Education and Welfare, Fiscal Division, Federal Sterilization Regulations, 42 CFR, part 441, Sub F, February 1979.

3. Position Paper on the Current Status of Federally-funded Sterilizations, Association of Planned Parenthood Physicians, February 1980.

4. *Voluntary Sterilization: Your right to know; Your right to choose.* New York, Association for Voluntary Sterilization, Inc, 1978.

5. Woodruff JD, Pauerstein CM: *The Fallopian Tube,* Baltimore, Williams and Wilkins, 1969, pp 347–351.

6. Savage D: The claim for wrongful conception. *J Reprod Med* 24:51, 1980.

7 Anesthesia for Tubal Sterilization

CHOICE OF ANESTHETIC TECHNIQUE FOR TUBAL STERILIZATION

Anesthesia for tubal sterilization may be local or general, and it may be administered by a trained anesthesiologist, a nurse-anesthetist, or by the surgeon himself. The determining factors which guide not only the choice of the anesthesia but also the method used are in part decided by which method of tubal sterilization has been chosen.

We have previously expressed our bias in favor of general anesthesia. Under certain circumstances (eg, respiratory infection) regional anesthesia administered by a trained anesthesiologist is acceptable for reasons of patient safety and comfort, as well as for surgeon comfort and overall satisfaction. It would at first seem preferable to use only local anesthesia under all circumstances and to use an anesthetic that can be administered by the surgeon, thereby reducing the need for additional trained personnel, supplies, equipment, and cost to the patient (or insurance carrier). However, such a universally applicable anesthesia method has not yet been devised and probably never will be found.

In our own short series, when local anesthesia was used with mini-laparotomy cases, we had grossly unsatisfactory experiences because heavy doses of analeptic agents and narcotics were required to achieve minimally acceptable patient cooperation, Pennfield's excellent results[1] and a similar report by Whitaker (personal communication, October 1979) notwithstanding. In several instances, the amount of these drugs exceeded that used by our anesthesiologist administering balanced general anesthesia. Furthermore, in this day of a litigationally sensitized public, we do not feel secure in taking the responsibility for being both the surgeon and anesthesiologist at the same time.

In tubal sterilization by means of the vaginal route, sufficient muscular relaxation is mandatory to prevent the operative field from becoming crowded with loops of bowel. This factor also makes the use of local anesthesia for VTS unacceptable.

Possibly in laparoscopy or mini-laparotomy cases, with certain selected patients and technically expert operators, local anesthesia can and should be used; therefore, it ought not be dismissed entirely.[2] However, Schonberg[3] and others express their preference for general over local anesthesia for other nontechnical but nonetheless important considerations: "Cultural factors come into play; these include one's expectations of operative discomfort, what degree of discomfort one is willing to accept, and the widespread knowledge that general anesthesia is readily available in this country (and especially in our community)."[3]

For our purposes and in our series, we elected to use general anesthesia because it allows for decreased operating time, improves surgical exposure and efficiency, avoids inadequate anesthesia with its mandatory use of large doses of analeptic or basal analgesic drugs, provides excellent patient acceptance, and increases patient safety by avoidance of compromises necessitated by inadequate local anesthesia.

PROCEDURES FOR ADMINISTRATION OF ANESTHESIA TO TUBAL STERILIZATION PATIENTS

The patients chosen for the vaginal tubal sterilization procedure, having been thoroughly screened for medical contraindications to general anesthesia, counseled, and examined at a suitable clinic facility prior to admission to the hospital or day-surgery center, arrive on the morning of the day of surgery with an empty stomach. If the patient has no allergies to analgesia-producing drugs, preoperative medication consisting of 50 mg meperidine hydrochloride, 25 mg promethazine hydrochloride, and 0.4 mg atropine sulfate is given intramuscularly one hour before surgery. When the patient arrives in the operating theater, an intravenous catheter is placed in her left hand or forearm, and lactated Ringer's solution in 5% dextrose in water is administered. Induction of anesthesia is accomplished with 10 ml of 2% sodium thiopental (200 mg) and immediately followed by 4 ml of fentanyl citrate (0.2 mg) and 3 ml of succinylcholine chloride (60 mg). The lungs are ventilated with 100% oxygen by face mask until muscular fasciculations are seen to stop. The vocal cords and trachea are then visualized with a laryngoscope and topically anesthetized with 4 ml of 4% lidocaine solution. Endotracheal intubation immediately follows with a suitable endotracheal tube. Anesthesia is maintained with nitrous oxide (4 L/min), oxygen (2 L/min), and 0.1% succinylcholine chloride IV drip as needed.

At the beginning of the closure of the colpotomy, the surgeon alerts the anesthesiologist, signaling an appropriate time to stop the muscle-relaxant drug (succinylcholine chloride). At the end of the surgical procedure, the nitrous oxide is turned off, the flow of oxygen increased to 4 L/min, and 1 ml of naloxone hydrochloride (0.4 mg) is given intravenously. After mucus has been suctioned from the oral cavity and good spontaneous ventilation has been reestablished, the patient is extubated. By this time she is usually awake and able to talk and move with little or no assistance from the operating table to the wheeled stretcher for transfer to the recovery room. There, humidified oxygen mist is administered by face tent at 4 L/min to obviate respiratory depression. When finally awake and alert (usually after 30 minutes), the patient is returned to her room and discharged to her own care later the same day.

To further ensure patient safety, a cardiac monitor displaying electrical heart activity on a cathode-ray tube is in constant use, and resuscitative equipment is available.[4]

CONTRAINDICATIONS TO GENERAL ANESTHESIA

Several factors contraindicate the use of general anesthesia including inability to intubate the patient, severe and unresponsive hypotensive or hypertensive episodes, development of malignant hyperthermia during anesthesia, unresponsive cardiac arrhythmias, marked anemia, generalized debilitating conditions, or preexisting febrile states.

The only anesthesia-related complication in the present series was a mild sore throat, presumably caused by the endotracheal tube.

REFERENCES

1. Pennfield AJ: *Female Sterilization by Mini-Laparotomy or Open Laparoscopy,* Baltimore, Urban and Schwarzenberg, 1980.
2. Ibid.
3. Schonberg I: (ltr to ed). *Obstet Gynecol News* 15:5, 1980.
4. Kurn J: Method of anesthesia for vaginal tubal sterilization: Personal communication, San Antonio, Texas, May 1980.

8 Preoperative Procedures

PREOPERATIVE REQUIREMENTS

Day Before Surgery

It is desirable for the patient to have taken a thorough shower or bath and have the pubic hair cut short (about ¼ in). Shaving of this tender area is neither necessary nor desirable since this practice may increase the risk of subsequent infection from colonization of the skin with pathogenic organisms. A laxative or, in the event of its failure, an enema is helpful to reduce the risk of rectal injury during the colpotomy incision.

The last meal should be no later than 10:00 PM and not even liquids should be taken after midnight. This simple precaution considerably reduces the risk of aspiration of food or fluids during and following surgery and may decrease postoperative nausea.

Day Of Surgery

The patient should arrive at the hospital no later than one hour prior to the scheduled time of surgery. A responsible adult must be available to transport her to the facility and, at the conclusion of the initial recuperative period, back to her home. Once at the hospital, final review of financial entitlements, operative permits, and all laboratory results are necessary; the chest roentgenograms, complete blood count, urinalysis, syphilis serologic test, Pap smear, and gonorrhea culture are reviewed.

Written preoperative and postoperative instructions are once again explained to the patient and, if possible, to her responsible adult escort. (See Chapter 5 and Appendix 3 for sample instructions.) The patient is then put to bed and given preoperative medications (see Chapter 7 on anesthesia), awaiting her turn at surgery.

INSTRUMENTS FOR VAGINAL TUBAL STERILIZATION

One of the major advantages of the vaginal approach to sterilization is the ready availability of instruments. These are inexpensive, standard in nomenclature, sturdy, and easily maintained by minimally trained technicians. For a list of instruments required for VTS refer to Table 8-1.

Table 8-1
Instruments for Vaginal Tubal Sterilization

---

1. Forceps: 1 Adson forceps, large, double-toothed (8 in)
   1 Bozeman (uterine packing) forceps (10 in)
   2 Ring forceps, long (8 in) (one curved and one straight)
   1 Magill endotracheal-tube–introducing forceps
   2 Allis forceps, blunted (8 in)

2. Clamps: 2 Hemostats, curved, small (5½ in)
   1 Hemostat, tonsil (used as ligature carrier) (7½ in)
   2 Heaney, curved (preferably Ballantine modification) hysterectomy clamps
   1 Babcock long clamp (9 in)

3. Needleholders: 1 Heaney-type (8 in) preferable, or 1 straight needleholder (8 in)

4. Retractors: 1 Sims retractor
   1 baby Deaver, narrow blade (¾ in)

5. Scissors: 1 Mayo straight scissors (for sutures) (7½ in)
   1 Mayo curved scissors (for dissecting) (7½ in)
   1 Metzenbaum scissors (8 in)

6. Suction: tubing (flexible) with metal tonsil-type handle and tip

7. Sutures: #1 black silk (60 in) for ties (Davis and Geck #1037–71 or similar)
   #1 chromic catgut (27 in) with small, heavy, taper needle (Ethicon #885 or similar)
   or polyglycolate suture (27 in) (Dexon-S 7248–61 with T19 taper needle)

8. Tenacula: 1 Lahey tenaculum, thyroid clamp (6 in)
   2 cervical tenacula, single tooth, long (10 in)

9. Weighted specula: 1 Auvard, short blade (2½ in) or Soonawallah combination speculum
   1 Auvard, long blade (5½ in) speculum

10. Special Instruments (optional):
    Hulka clip applicator (R. Wolf Instrument Co.) and spring-loaded clips and/or Yoon Band applicator (J. Eder Instrument Co.) and silicone elastic bands

11. Towels, lithotomy drape, towel clips (5½ in), standard instrument table and tray (for placing instruments on lap)

12. Laryngoscope, Foregger with #2 Miller blade (6 in)

13. IV fluids: dextrose 5%, lactated Ringer's solution, 1000 ml (Abbott)

14. IV administration set, nonvented, product #1857 (Abbott)

15. Endotracheal tube 7.5: (Rusch)

16. Forescope monitor: (Foregger)

17. Defibrillator: (Burdick)

18. Ambu bag: (Ohio Medical)

19. Respiration unit: (Bennet) Model PR-2

20. Anesthesia machine, Foretrend (Foregger) with enflurane, halothane, pentrane, nitrous oxide, and oxygen

21. Ventilator, Ventimeter: Air Shield

22. Skin prep tray, disposable (povidone-iodine) product #212 (Abbott)

POSITIONING AND OPERATING ROOM PREPARATION

For the positioning of personnel and equipment in the operating room see Figure 8-1.

Positioning

The patient is positioned in the middle of the table with her buttocks at the break. The right arm is folded across the chest and immobilized by a fold of the patient's gown.

General endotracheal (or regional) anesthesia (see Chapter 7) is induced after starting an intravenous infusion (in the left hand or

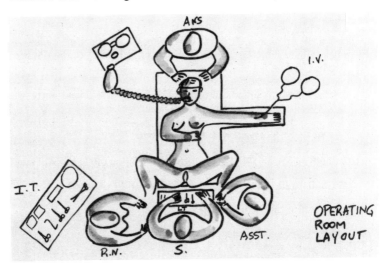

Figure 8-1 Operating room layout. ANS = anesthesiologist, ASST = surgical assistant, IT = instrument table, LT = lap tray for instruments, RN = instrument nurse, S = surgeon (seated).

wrist, if possible). Once anesthesia has been induced, the patient is placed in a modified dorsal lithotomy position with moderate extension of the knees and flexion of the thighs. The buttocks should slightly overhang the edge of the table (Figure 8-2). One to three degrees of Trendelenburg position is desirable to aid in allowing the viscera to fall away from the operative field.

Preparation

The patient had previously been instructed to clip the labial hair to 1/8 to 1/4 in (shaving the labia and pubis proved unnecessary). The pubis and vagina are then scrubbed with povidone-iodine soap solution for five minutes (by clock) and a pool of povidone-iodine aqueous solution is left in the vagina. The perineum is then draped with towels over which a lithotomy drape covers buttocks, legs, stirrup posts, and abdomen (thus providing standard double-thickness draping).

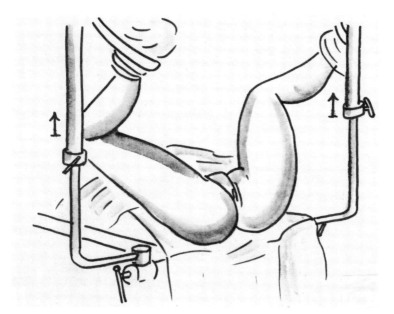

Figure 8-2 Positioning of patient for vaginal tubal sterilization.

9 Operative Technique

ENTERING THE CUL-DE-SAC

A careful pelvic examination is performed to determine freedom of the cul-de-sac, mobility of the uterus, and absence of adnexal or other pelvic pathology. During this pelvic examination an attempt is made to retrovert the uterus. Occasionally, an intrauterine instrument is required to assist in this maneuver (Figure 9-1).

A short-bladed (2½ in) Auvard speculum is placed against the posterior vaginal wall, the cervix is visualized, and the posterior lip is grasped with a Lahey thyroid tenaculum. This clamp then is moved gently back and forth to identify the cul-de-sac bulge. Two Allis clamps are placed on the cul-de-sac vaginal mucosa behind the cervix and between the uterosacral ligaments at their decussation point. The axis of the clamps is set at right angles to the mucosal rugae. The placement of these clamps is critical to opening the cul-de-sac at the optimal point for sufficient lateral exposure. The cervix is then elevated smartly to provide mucosal tension. The opening of the cul-de-sac is accomplished with a single transverse "bold snip"[1] with curved Mayo scissors, attempting to cut the mucosa and peritoneum

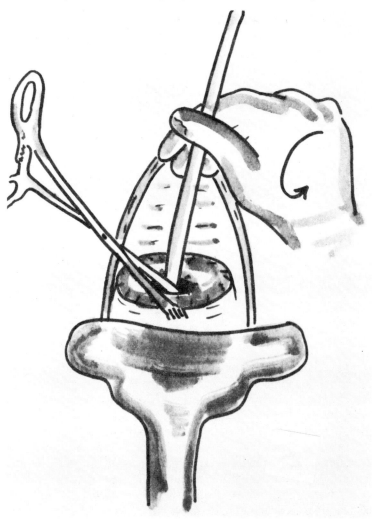

Figure 9-1   Initial maneuver to retrovert the uterus.

simultaneously by upward traction on the cervix and downward pressure on the speculum (Figures 9-2, 9-3). If the initial cut fails to enter the peritoneal cavity, care must be taken to proceed in the right

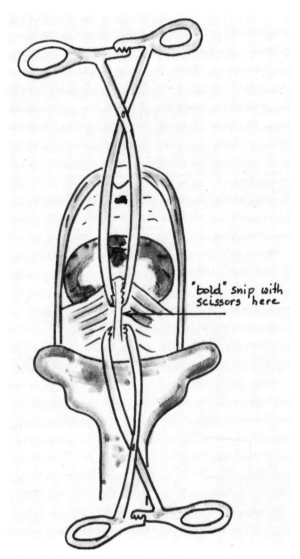

"bold" snip with scissors here

Figure 9-2 Opening the posterior vaginal cul-de-sac A.

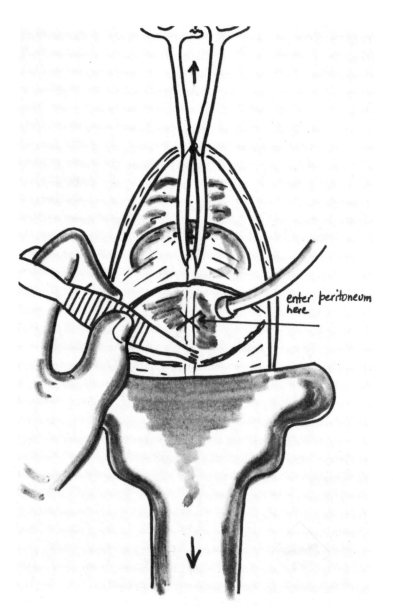

enter peritoneum here

Figure 9-3 Opening the posterior vaginal cul-de-sac B.

plane; misdirected dissection anteriorly tunnels into the posterior uterine wall or posteriorly into the perirectal space or the rectum, both leading to annoying and excessive bleeding (the ominous clue that one is in the wrong place). The incision is widened laterally either by forcibly withdrawing the spread blades of the scissors, or digitally. The uterosacral ligaments are not cut.

EXPOSURE OF THE FALLOPIAN TUBES

A long-bladed (5½ in) Auvard speculum is now substituted for the short speculum and placed within the peritoneal cul-de-sac. The Lahey tenaculum is repositioned to include the peritoneal reflection in the posterior jaw, thereby shortening the cul-de-sac peritoneum by traction and helping to retrovert the uterus into the incision. A narrow (¾ in) baby Deaver retractor is then placed alternately in the peritoneal angles. The fallopian tube may now spontaneously appear at the incisional angle. If the tube has not been visualized by this time, the following maneuvers are tried in turn:

1. Introduce a longitudinally folded 4 x 4 in gauze sponge held in a straight ring forceps as far laterally and anteriorly as possible, and sweep medially and inferiorly. Repeated sweeps are sometimes necessary before visualization is obtained.
2. "Go fishing" blindly with the ring or Magill forceps in the most promising areas to bring the tube and/or ovary into view (Figure 9-4).
3. Firmly retrovert the uterine fundus into the incision by the following maneuvers:
   a. Introduce a Hegar dilator or closed Bozeman uterine dressing forceps into the uterine cavity, manipulating the uterine fundus posteriorly and contralaterally into the incision until the tube or ovary is visualized (see Figure 9-1).
   b. Using two single-tooth tenacula and taking wide "bites" into the posterior myometrium, "walk" the uterine fundus into acute retroflexion and contralaterally until visualization is obtained. Caution:

gentle traction on these tenacula is mandatory; otherwise, vigorously bleeding lacerations will be produced.
4. Frequently the ovary is visualized before the tube. In

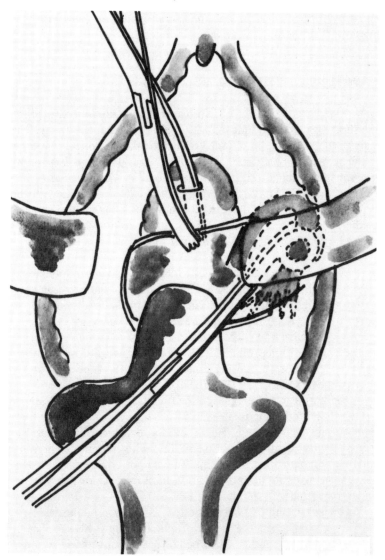

Figure 9-4 Mobilizing the fallopian tube.

this case, traction on the ovary will nearly always bring the tube, or a portion thereof, into the visual field. Avoid lacerating the ovarian capsule by using only *incompletely* closed ring or Magill forceps. The tube can now be grasped and the fimbriated end "walked" into the field. Failing this, a segmental tubal resection (Pomeroy procedure) is carried out if further mobilization is not possible.

5. Abandon the colpotomy approach after a *reasonable* trial at visualization. Close the colpotomy incision and switch to the mini-laparotomy technique. Note: if the tubes cannot be seen from behind, they *must* be seen from the front.

It was interesting for us to note that, as we gained experience and expertise, we were able to determine with dispatch how long to persist in attempting to find the tubes by these various maneuvers and to proceed quite rapidly from the least difficult to the more technically involved methods; we also accepted defeat at these attempts without as much delay, and moved to mini-laparotomy when failure appeared to be inevitable.

MANAGEMENT OF THE TUBES

To assure that an adequate length of tube can be resected, the Heaney clamp must be placed close to the ovary and *include* the fimbria ovarica. We prefer a modified Kroener fimbriectomy technique.[2] Clamp the tube with a curved Heaney clamp, amputate the fimbriated infundibular end, and free-tie with a single ligature of #1 black silk placed immediately behind the clamp and "snugged" down as the clamp is removed (Figures 9-5, 9-6). Segmental resection of the tube (Pomeroy) is used only when visualization of the infundibulum is not possible. We use a #0 chromic-catgut-suture-ligature, taking care to perforate only the mesosalpinx but not the tube itself. Amputate the "knuckle" of the tube and send it to the laboratory for frozen-section pathologic confirmation if there is any question that the specimen is indeed a portion of the fallopian tube (Figures 9-7, 9-9). The surgical anatomy of the adnexa referable to the Kroener and Pomeroy techniques of tubal resection is illustrated in Figures 9-8 and 9-9.

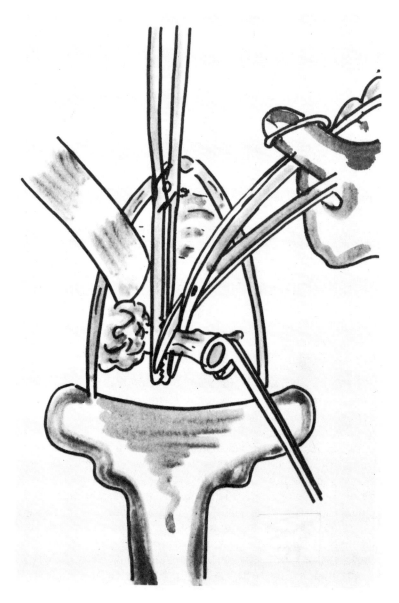

Figure 9-5 Amputation of the fimbriated end of the tube (the Kroener technique)

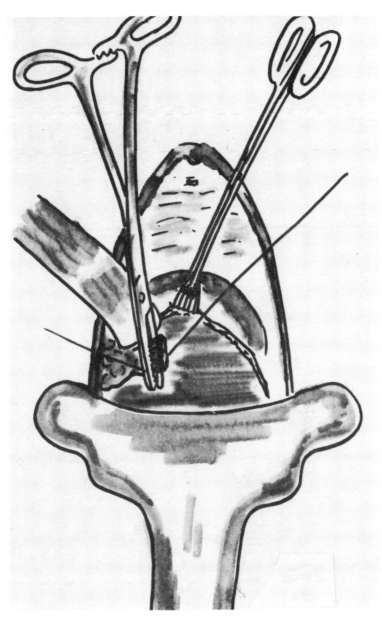

Figure 9-6 Ligating the tube (the Kroener technique)

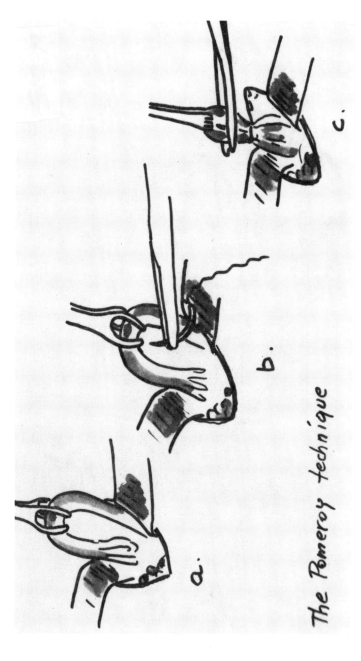

The Pomeroy technique

Figure 9-7 The Pomeroy technique of tubal resection

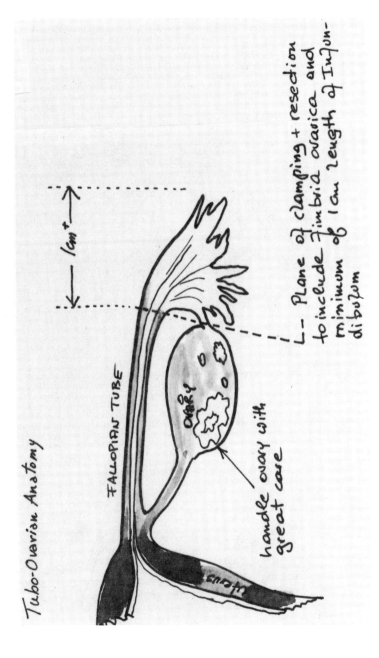

Figure 9-8 Surgical anatomy concerned with the Kroener technique

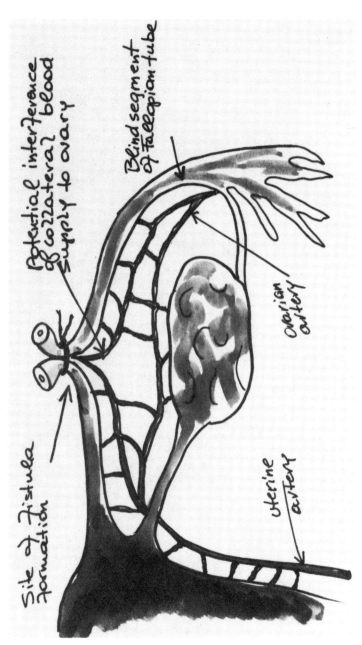

Potential interference of collateral blood supply to ovary

Blind segment of fallopian tube

Site of fistula formation

ovarian artery

uterine artery

Figure 9-9 Surgical anatomy concerned with the Pomeroy technique

CLOSURE

Closure is accomplished with a running, nonlocking suture of #1 chromic catgut or preferably, #0 polyglycolate suture on a short, stout taper needle. The suture is begun to the patient's left and posteriorly, and includes, in turn, mucosa, posterior, and then anterior peritoneal reflections, and mucosa; it is started just lateral to the left incisional angle (Figure 9-10). The long-bladed speculum is

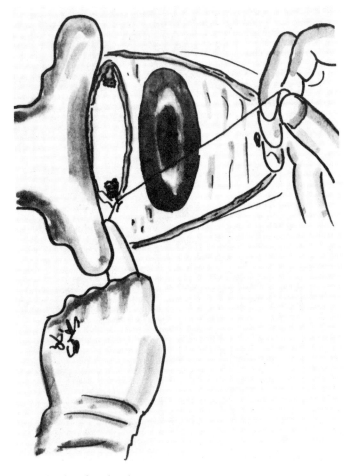

Figure 9-10   Starting the closure

left in place until the suture is tied, as is the Lahey tenaculum. Exposure of the angle is facilitated by pushing the jaws of the Lahey

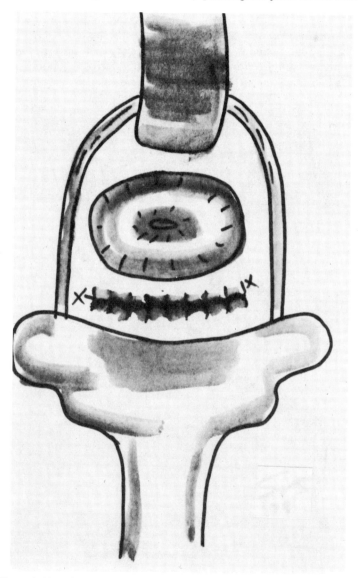

Figure 9-11 Closure complete

tenaculum as far as possible toward the patient's right. The Lahey tenaculum is then removed and the short-bladed Auvard speculum replaced on the posterior vaginal wall. The nonlocking suture is run from the patient's left to right, including the dead space at the incisional angles and between mucosa and peritoneum posteriorly. If indicated, a modified enterocele repair may now be performed by shortening and partially obliterating the peritoneum of the pouch of Douglas.

Approximating the vaginal mucosa only, without closing the peritoneum, is also acceptable. Occasionally, an "obliteration suture," approximating a portion of the incisional vaginal mucosa to the mucosal reflection over the posterior lip of the cervix, is advantageous for hemostasis at the tenaculum site. The running ligature is completed and tied just lateral to the right angle of the incision. No packs or drains are used (Figure 9-11).

REFERENCES

1. Purandare VN: Evaluation of operative methods for female sterilization, Conference on Family Planning and Biology of Reproduction. Bombay, India, March 3-8, 1969.

2. Kroener WF, Jr: Surgical sterilization by fimbriectomy. *Am J Obstet Gynecol* 104:247, 1969.

10 Postoperative Period

INITIAL (FIRST SIX HOURS IN FACILITY)

The patient is moved from the operating theater to the recovery room where she is observed until her vital signs have stabilized and she is fully awake (usually 20 to 30 minutes). She is then transferred to the surgical floor for four to six hours (or until the end of the working day). Included in the usual postoperative orders are the following: diet conforming to the patient's wishes and tolerances, as well as the permission to ambulate as she is able; 60 mg codeine sulfate or 50 mg meperidine hydrochloride, given either by mouth or intramuscular injection (strong analgesics such as these are usually required no more than twice during the postoperative period). Prochlorperazine or thiethylperazine, 10 mg intramuscularly, is required occasionally, if at all, for antiemesis in

79

the early postoperative period, usually just after emergence from anesthesia.

The patient may be dismissed from the day-surgery unit when she is observed to be fully awake, her vital signs are stabilized for an appropriate length of time, and she experiences no significant vaginal bleeding, especially after assuming the upright position. The presence of a responsible person to accompany the patient from the facility is mandatory. Provision for regular, inpatient admission must be available at any time during the postoperative period.

INTERMEDIATE (SIX HOURS TO FOURTEEN DAYS)

The patient is advised to limit her activities for 24 hours. She is told that pelvic discomfort may persist for the first 48 hours postoperatively. Penile-vaginal intercourse, douching, and the use of tampons are discouraged for two weeks postoperatively. Recognizing that social pressures and the sudden alteration of life-style imposed by the proscription of penile-vaginal intercourse may be difficult for many patients to carry out, we advise our patients during the immediate postoperative period that alternate methods of sexual expression are definitely acceptable. By that advice, we mean to make a positive suggestion that other areas of sexuality and physical contact are appropriate and ought to be explored while leaving the operative site undisturbed for healing.

The patient is instructed verbally and in writing to contact the surgeon if any of the following occur: significant vaginal bleeding, persistent or foul discharge, fever of 100.4°F (38°C) or higher, or abdominal pain with or without distention. In giving the patient postoperative instructions, we have found the acronym "Call For Help"[1] a useful memory device for the patient's use. The first letter of each of the three words stands for a danger sign which ought to be reported: cramps, fever or foul discharge, hemorrhage (See Appendix 3 for example of instruction sheet).

LATE (FOURTEEN DAYS AND BEYOND)

The patient is asked to return for abdominal and pelvic examination (both bimanual and speculum) two weeks postoperatively.

Because of the potential problem of concomitant luteal phase pregnancy, *a urine pregnancy test is performed routinely at this time.*

The patient is counseled on follow-up about any gynecologic problems uncovered either during preoperative evaluation or the surgical procedure, and is informed of the pathologic findings on the tissue submitted for examination at surgery.

REFERENCES

1. Bell E: *Instructions to Postoperative Patients,* Reproductive Services, Inc, San Antonio, Texas, 1980.

11 Clinical Experience with Tubal Sterilization

DISCUSSION OF TUBAL STERILIZATION EXPERIENCE

We evaluated the first 500 procedures. See Table 11-1.

Colpotubal-Kroener procedures were performed in 92.6% of our cases. Mini-laparotomies for impaired vaginal approach were required only six times (1.2%): once for an unmobilized, unruptured, ectopic pregnancy requiring salpingectomy, and once for a large dermoid cyst of one ovary treated by salpingo-oophorectomy in a grossly obese woman. Two elective mini-laparotomies were managed on the same outpatient regimen as VTS without additional complications. There were four postoperative pregnancies (0.8%), two of them luteal phase gestations. The only failure to resect a tube, a unilateral Pomeroy ligation, subsequently was found to be a tubal occlusion demonstrated by salpingogram.

Table 11-1
Clinical Experiences with 500 Vaginal Tubal Sterilizations

Type	Number	%	
Colpoceliotomy			
Bilateral Kroener	463	92.6	
Bilateral Pomeroy	1	0.2	
Mixed type	24	4.8	
For single remaining tube (all Kroener)	4	0.8	
Mini-laparotomy			
Elective	2	0.4	
For impaired vaginal approach	6	1.2	
	500	100.0%	
Complications	Number	%	
Major			
Deaths	0	0.0	
Failures (postoperative pregnancies	2	0.4	0.8% total
Luteal phase pregnancies	2	0.4	pregnancies
Failure to resect tubes	1	0.2	
Pelvic inflammatory disease (PID)	7	1.4	2.0% total
PID with tubo-ovarian abscess	3	0.6	infectious morbidity
Minor			
Incisional bleeding	13	2.6	
Persistent vaginal granulations	18	3.6	
Abdominal pain without evidence of PID	8	1.6	
Anesthetic complications	1	0.2	
Bowel injury	0	0.0	
Cystitis	2	0.4	
Dyspareunia	0	0.0	
Total	57	11.4	
Hospitalization for treatment of complications	8	1.6	
Surgery required for treatment of complications	6	1.2	

Major complications were primarily infectious in nature. Pelvic inflammatory disease (PID), defined as fever, pain, leukocytosis, and elevated sedimentation rate, occurred in seven cases (1.4%), only two of which required inpatient, antibiotic therapy. PID with tubo-ovarian abscess occurred three times (0.6%), all requiring surgical drainage. The total infectious morbidity was 2.0%.

Minor complications included vaginal-incisional bleeding which occurred in thirteen cases (2.6%). No one became anemic (less than 10 g hemoglobin) and only two required hospitalization for operating room resuture. Persistent vaginal granulations with leukorrhea occurred 18 times (3.6%). Abdominal pain without evidence of PID was seen in eight cases (1.6%). The only anesthetic complication was one case of a sore throat for more that 24 hours postoperatively.

MANAGEMENT AND PREVENTION OF SOME POSTOPERATIVE COMPLICATIONS

Pelvic Inflammatory Disease (PID)

Most of these complications subsided promptly and completely with oral antibiotics and "pelvic rest" without hospitalization. Ampicillin was usually the first-choice drug, barring patient allergy, but the cephalosporins and tetracyclines seemed equally effective. A seven-day course was prescribed, either with or without analgesics. A follow-up visit to confirm resolution of the inflammation is mandatory. If the patient was using an IUD, it should have been removed at least one menstrual cycle prior to tubal surgery to allow for endometrial healing. Experience in our community[1] with laparoscopic tubal sterilizations has led us to believe that performing tubal ligation with the IUD in place leads to a greater risk of postoperative infection.

PID With Tubo-Ovarian Abscess

This major and most vexing problem occurred in only three (0.6%) of our patients but was the most serious complication encountered. The organisms involved were mixed, including anaerobes

85

(a positive culture in one patient and gross surgical findings in the others), and were presumably inoculated into the pelvis from the vagina.

Preoperative diagnosis was based upon failure of clinical response to adequate single or combination courses of antibiotics. Usually there was little or no fever and only mild to moderate toxicity. Persistent unilateral pain was pathognomonic. Total abdominal hysterectomy with bilateral salpingo-oophorectomy may be the procedure of choice, but unilateral salpingo-oophorectomy or rectal or vaginal drainage may at times be acceptable.[2,3] Optimal antibiotic coverage with any surgical approach is mandatory.

The critical reader may well ask why, if these investigators consider VTS as their preferred method, it has not generally enjoyed more enthusiastic acceptance? As we see it, there is but one major underlying reason for this reluctance: the unfounded fear of infection. It is suspected that following other vaginal procedures, such as vaginal hysterectomy with or without colpoplasty, as many as 40% of patients will have some infectious morbidity.[4] By inference, VTS also is suspected of being associated with a high postoperative infection-risk. To evaluate the validity of this fear, one must differentiate between VTS and vaginal surgery performed in conjunction with underlying disease processes (eg, endometriosis, adenomyosis, chronic pelvic peritonitis). Tissue-plane dissection associated with plastic repair versus the clean, planned, and simple vaginal tubal sterilization may be responsible for such a high infection rate. These are not comparable operative procedures, yet they have all been considered together, thus discrediting the vaginal route to permanent sterilization.

Another and probably equally important source of confusion arises out of the lack of uniformity of terms. PID is a "catch-all" category including many diseases, such as pelvic cellulitis, pelvic abscess, salpingitis, and oophoritis, and each of these has its own course ranging from mild to severe. Another factor relating to vaginal surgery and infection is the definitely adverse association of a concomitantly performed termination of pregnancy.[5] If VTS is performed as an interval procedure, this cause of infection is avoided.

Our 1.6% rate of infection compares well with Miesfeld's 1.2%,[6] Shepard's review rate of 1.5% to 2.5%,[7] and Wortman and Pietrow's review rate of 2.5%.[8] Overall, these are low rates of infection comparing favorably with rates for other gynecologic surgery. Admittedly, the postoperative infection rate in laparoscopically performed tubal sterilization is lower than that in vaginally performed surgery. In a study of laparoscopically performed tubal sterilizations, done in our community under general anesthesia on an outpatient basis, we found the pelvic infection rate to be 0.93%.[1] However, the trade-off with other major complications accompanying laparoscopic procedures, such as bowel lacerations, blood vessel injury, possibly burns to adjacent structures, etc, more than balances the scales.

In our experience, most pelvic infections (1.8% of 2.0% total) occurred in the form of cellulitis, a readily treated form of infection. Seven patients (1.4%) required only oral antibiotics on an outpatient basis, and only three women (0.6%) needed parenteral antibiotic therapy in the hospital. Tubo-ovarian abscess occurred infrequently (0.6%).

The above-cited literature as well as Gananagarangasam's summary[2] makes *no distinction* among these varying forms of pelvic infection, thereby inducing apprehension and rejection of the vaginal approach, an undeserved bias.

With regard to the treatment of pelvic abscess with associated pelvic peritonitis, this type of pelvic sepsis requires total abdominal hysterectomy and bilateral salpingo-oophorectomy together with anaerobic antibiotic coverage. Well-demarcated, indolent infection involving the distal tube may be treated effectively by unilateral adnexal resection with good antibiotic coverage. Colpotomy drainage is probably indicated only in cases of long-standing pelvic abscesses pointing in the cul-de-sac, or when the surgery is performed under inadequate conditions where laparotomy and pelvic "clean-out" would be dangerous because of limited facilities.

It is a common belief among surgeons that the patient's "constitutional factors" are at least in part responsible for postoperative complications like wound dehiscence and infection. Such vague conditions as poor nutrition, poor "protoplasm", and poor hygiene have all been blamed. It stands to reason that gross malnutrition, both *underweight and overweight*, a diet lacking in protein, and poor body hygiene resulting in intertriginous skin infestations or infections could be associated with poor postoperative results. However, proof of this assertion based on more than anecdotes or experiences in Nazi Germany concentration camps is hard to obtain. The role played by malnutrition in systemic disease, however, is definitely clearer. Vitamin deficiencies, hormone dysfunction, protein and mineral deficiencies are all directly related to a state of poor wound healing and to a breakdown of the natural host resistance, either through enzyme or coenzyme failure or poor antibody formation.[9]

In light of the foregoing ill-defined factors, we examined all pertinent variables of those patients who had developed postoperative complications. There appeared to be no causal relationship between those cases where difficulty of exposure was encountered or where the ovarian capsule was inadvertently ruptured during the attempt to mobilize the fallopian tubes, and postoperative infections or troublesome granulations. There remain only "constitutional factors" to blame for these rare, yet troublesome, complications.

Pelvic Pain Without Evidence of PID

Postoperative pain, sometimes unilateral, is occasionally noted to follow all types of tubal sterilization. It occurred in 1.6% of our patients and has also been reported by others.[1,7,8,10] Significantly *absent* are persistent fever, leukocytosis, and elevated sedimentation rate. Abdominal muscle guarding has frequently been noted and can even be confused with the presence of a mass. Most patients in our series improved on analgesics and pelvic rest alone. Many were treated with antibiotics empirically; all followed a benign clinical course.

The etiology of this syndrome at the present time is unclear and may be related to inflammatory, vascular, neurogenic, or psychogenic causes. One might assume that, following posterior colpotomy, a certain number of patients would complain of dyspareunia for psychosexual reasons. This indeed has been reported by some investigators.[10,20] As yet, we have not observed this occurrence in our series; one can only speculate as to the absence of this complaint. Careful preoperative counseling, gentle operative technique, and a transient population may play a significant role.

Incisional Bleeding

With only one exception, this complication occurred 10 to 14 days postoperatively. The bleeding site usually was along part or all of the colpotomy incision and frequently was from the left angle alone. If there was venous oozing, control was usually attained by packing with a pledget of oxidized cellulose moistened with Monsel's solution (ferric subsulfate). If the bleeding was brisk and arterial in origin, one or more figure-of-eight sutures of #1 chromic catgut gave prompt control. In only two cases was operating room resuture of the entire incision required. Since we changed to a nonlocking closure of the colpotomy incision, adequate hemostasis has been obtained and no cases of delayed bleeding have occurred.

Persistent Vaginal Granulations

Complaints of foul, sometimes watery or bloody, vaginal discharge after ten days postoperatively are usually due to subacutely infected granulations of the suture line (proud flesh). Debridement of the granulations and remaining suture material plus cauterization with silver nitrate applicators (and ferric subsulfate solution if desired) clears the problem promptly. Since using a nonlocking colpotomy closure with polyglycolic acid suture material, we have not encountered this problem.

Failure of Pregnancy Prevention

Pregnancies occurring may be classified as preventable and nonpreventable.

Actually or potentially preventable pregnancies may be due to ligation of structures other than the tube, such as the round ligament or varicose veins; inappropriate use of suture materials, such as absorbable sutures in fimbriectomies or nonabsorbable sutures in segmental resections; and failure to recognize accessory ostia of the tube or failure to include the fimbria ovarica in the ligature in fimbriectomy.

Nonpreventable pregnancies may result from subsequent development of tuboperitoneal fistulae (either mini-fimbriae or microscopic) or development of an ectopic tubal pregnancy in the distal, blind (occluded) segment of the tube. The latter requires at least a microscopic tubal fistula to allow for the escape of spermatozoa into the peritoneal cavity with subsequent entrapment of a fertilized ovum in the distal tube.[11] Loffer and Laufe[12] report a 15:1 intrauterine ectopic pregnancy rate within two years of the original surgery and a 1:1 ratio thereafter up to four years. Miesfeld[5] reports a very high pregnancy rate of 2.4%. Metz[13] reports a 1.8% pregnancy rate in 388 bilateral fimbriectomies, of which 131 were done by the vaginal route; use of catgut suture material and failure to include an adequate distal segment of tube to include the fimbria ovarica probably were to blame. Gibbons[14] reports failures in relation to the choice of the original tubal closure procedures, as previously reported in Table 2-5. Tatum and Schmidt[15] reported the lowest incidence of ectopic pregnancy to occur after tubal sterilization by the vaginal route. This is borne out in our series where, as yet, we have had none.

The goal, of course, is to perform the tubal sterilization in the manner least likely to produce a failure; however, the patient is so counseled that she is willing to accept possible failure as an unavoidable risk to this procedure. VTS is still at least ten times more effective in preventing pregnancy than the best present reversible method, ie, oral contraceptives. We feel that the responsibility of accepting risk lies with the *patient*, as long as she has been fully informed of these chances of inherent failure.

Menstrual Timing for Tubal Sterilization Surgery

We are in full agreement with others[16,17] that tubal sterilization should be performed during the proliferative phase of the menstrual cycle in order to avoid allowing luteal phase gestation to become a complication of the surgery. Unfortunately, the problem cannot be solved by optimal timing of the procedure alone. Factors relative to menstrual timing which might frustrate the surgeon's attempts to prevent pregnancy are post-pill amenorrhea, creating an uncertain time of ovulation; failure of spermicide or barrier method immediately preoperatively; complete omission of contraception because of psychological factors; misunderstanding on the part of the patient; or the often inevitable "administrative mistakes."

Alternate approaches to avoid this last-minute failure of contraception include continuing the patient who is already on oral contraceptives (provided they are 50 μg or less in estrogen content) through the time of her surgical procedure, providing her with spermicidal foam and/or condoms, or advising her to abstain from vaginal sexual intercourse from the time of counseling until two weeks postoperatively.

Although obviously desirable, timing of tubal surgery is probably not a controllable factor with patients funded by social welfare. It therefore becomes mandatory to make every effort at early pregnancy detection by performing a pregnancy test on each patient at the time of her two-week postoperative checkup. Fortunately, the sensitivity of the presently available urinary pregnancy test allows for the detection of a four-to-five-week gestation. If the visit is timed according to the outlined protocol (Chapter 5), this time interval

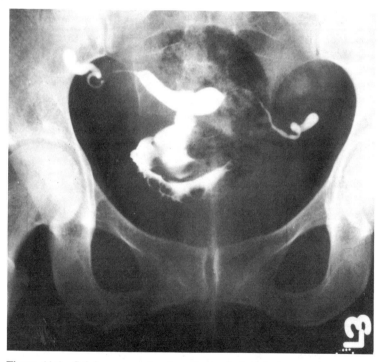

Figure 11-1 Salpingogram showing distal tubal occlusion as a result of a Kroener fimbriectomy. This patient had a luteal phase pregnancy at the time of VTS and elected to terminate the pregnancy. This study was performed six weeks after abortion.

should equal or be exceeded by the average surgery-to-checkup interval. Appropriate action may then be instituted at the earliest time.

In the event of a pregnancy occurring shortly after the sterilization procedure, one must document the existing status of the fallopian tubes after definitive management of this pregnancy. Appropriate counseling will allow the patient to express her desire for either subsequent obstetric delivery or interruption of the pregnancy. Such documentation is best obtained by the performance of a hysterosalpingogram. If both tubes are found to be occluded, a luteal phase pregnancy apparently caused the failure, and no further intervention needs to be made. In Figure 11-1 such an event is clearly demonstrated. If, however, tubal patency is apparent on the roentgenogram, a choice of either repeat tubal sterilization at no cost to the patient or hysterectomy should be offered that patient. This reoperation is best performed via laparotomy to allow maximal inspection of the tubes in order to elucidate the cause of the failure.

LONG-TERM FOLLOW-UP

In order to obtain a clear picture of the effectiveness of tubal sterilization through the vagina and determine the failure (pregnancy and other long-term complications) rate, a yearly inquiry over a period of at least five years is needed. As stated above, most failures will have occurred by the first postoperative year (as did our two). After two years, very few pregnancies have been reported, although cases have been cited in the literature up to 56 months.[12] We have established a five-year follow-up and intend to report our results after that time. With a largely transient population, many of whom are social-welfare recipients, the drop-out rate for follow-ups is expected to exceed 50%.

Post–Tubal-Ligation Syndrome

Much discussion has appeared in the literature, primarily anecdotally, about the existence of this entity. Unfortunately, there have been few controlled or prospective studies. Evaluation of the available results has been only subjective.

The major elements include menstrual irregularity (in terms of timing and character of flow), pelvic pain or pressure, and need for subsequent surgery. Additional aspects of the clinical situation include regret at having been sterilized, a general feeling of ill health, and a decreased satisfaction with sex.

Psychological biases in either patient or physician, aging, disruption of hypothalamic-pituitary-ovarian axis, ovarian dysfunction (vascular or neurogenic), pelvic congestion, prostaglandin excess, torsion of the distal tubal segment, and microspasm or microemboli in the ovarian circulation have all been blamed for this ill-defined condition.

Recent prospective studies[19,20] have failed to show any validity to this entity. Physicians who perform tubal sterilization are thus advised not to influence their patients adversely with overly detailed and pessimistic discussions of potential postoperative changes.

REFERENCES

1. Saidi M, Locke WE: Laparoscopic tubal sterilization in unselected outpatients. *Texas Med* 74:55, 1978.

2. Gananagarangasam JB: Colpotomy sterilization. *Ceylon Med* 22:196, 1976.

3. Berger GS, Keith L: Culdotomy for female sterilization. *Int Surg* 62:72, 1977.

4. Sweet RL: *Obstet Gynecol Annual* Vol 9, New York, Appleton, Century, Crofts, 1980.

5. Miesfeld RR, Giarratou RC, Moyers TG: Vaginal tubal ligation–is infection a significant risk? *Am J Obstet Gynecol* 137:183, 1980.

6. Ibid.

7. Shepard MK: Female contraceptive sterilization. *Obstet Gynecol Surv* 29:739, 1974.

8. Wortman J, Pietrow PT: Sterilization: Colpotomy—the vaginal approach. Population Report Series C #3, Washington University, 1973.

9. Madden TW: Wound healing; biologic and clinical features. In Sabiston DC (ed):*Davis-Christopher Textbook of Surgery; The Biologic Basis of Modern Surgical Practice, Tenth Edition,* Philadelphia, WB Saunders Co, 1972, p 249-271.

10. Yutzpe AA, Anderson RJ, Cohen NP, et al: A review of 1035 tubal sterilizations by posterior colpotomy under local anesthesia or by laparoscopy. *J Reprod Med* 13:106, 1974.

11. Metz KGP, Mastroianni L: Tubal pregnancy subsequent to transperitoneal migration of spermatozoa. *Obstet Gynecol Surv* [Suppl] 34:554, 1979.

12. Loffer F, Laufe L: Presentations at Centennial Conference on Voluntary Female Sterilization. Monterey, California, June 12, 1980.

13. Metz KGP: Failures following fimbriectomy. *Fertil Steril* 28:66, 1977.

14. Gibbons W: Presentation at Centennial Conference on Voluntary Female Sterilization. Monterey, California, June 12, 1980.

15. Tatum HT, Schmidt FH: Contraceptive sterilization practices and extrauterine pregnancy: A realistic perspective. *Fertil Steril* 28:407, 1977.

16. Whitaker KF: *Mini-laparotomy Protocol.* Nashville, Planned Parenthood Association of Nashville, 1979.

17. Pennfield AJ: *Female Sterilization by Mini-Laparotomy or Open Laparoscopy.* Baltimore, Urban and Schwarzenberg, 1980.

18. U.C.G.-Slide Test; Princeton Laboratory Products. Wampole Laboratories, Cranbury, New Jersey. Sensi-tex; Roche Diagnostics, Hoffmann-La-Roche, Nutley, New Jersey.

19. Levinson CJ: Presentation at Centennial Conference on Voluntary Female Sterilization. Monterey, California, June 12, 1980.

20. Rioux JE: Late complications of female sterilizations: A review of the literature and a proposal for further research. *J Reprod Med* 19:329, 1977.

12   Lessons Learned and Conclusions

From our clinical experience with 500 VTS, we learned six major lessons, summarized in Table 12-1.

Table 12-1
Lessons Learned

Lesson 1	VTS is easy to perform for a regularly trained surgeon with standard instruments.
Lesson 2	Contraindications must be heeded.
Lesson 3	General anesthesia is an advantage.
Lesson 4	Concomitant dilation and curettage is not required.
Lesson 5	Intraoperative warning signs must be heeded, without premature abandonment of the vaginal route.
Lesson 6	The procedure of choice must be fitted to the individual's needs, not vice versa.

Lesson 1: VTS proved to be a procedure easily mastered by trained surgeons, gynecologists, and family practitioners. It can be readily performed in an ordinary operating theater or a free-standing clinic using only the usually available assistants, equipment, and instruments.

Lesson 2: There are definite contraindications to the vaginal route to tubal sterilization. This is not a procedure universally applicable to everyone desiring permanent contraception. These contraindications are either *absolute* and *must* be observed or *relative* and *should* be followed. Active or recurrent pelvic inflammatory disease (PID); a blocked cul-de-sac, either from infections, adhesions, or endometriosis; an enlarged uterus greater than eight weeks gestational size from recent pregnancy, leiomyomata, adenomyosis, or a definite bleeding disorder, present absolute contraindications.

The presence of an IUD could be associated with a low-grade salpingitis which might flare up following tubal surgery (see Chapter 11, PID). A patient on oral contraceptive pills with greater than 50μg estrogen content reportedly is at a higher risk of subsequent thromboembolism.[1,2] The patient with obesity of greater than 20% over the average[3] presents technical difficulties to surgery via the vaginal route (see Chapter 11, Constitutional factors). The presence of other genital disease conditions (eg, endometriosis, tubo-ovarian disease, possibly congenital malformations) might interfere with ready exposure through the cul-de-sac, as do a deep or narrow vagina, high uterine suspension either from adhesions or operations, and nulliparity. All of these present *relative contraindications* and may allow only an attempt at VTS by a surgeon who must subsequently admit the need for mini-laparotomy or even rejection of the surgical approach to permanent contraception.

Lesson 3 General anesthesia has provided speed and efficiency in operations in this series. Rather than introducing hazards or complications,[4] it has helped us achieve excellent relaxation in totally cooperative patients whose physiological responses were predictable and readily controllable.

Lesson 4 During the first 400 cases in this series, a dilation and curettage was performed on each patient just prior to the VTS to interrupt any potentially coexisting intrauterine pregnancy. Since we encountered none, we elected to abandon this procedure as unnecessary and concentrated on careful counseling of the preoperative patient in preventing any last-minute pregnancy from occurring. Since curettage can only diagnose and interrupt an already implanted intrauterine pregnancy, our two luteal-phase pregnancies were probably still intratubal in location and therefore beyond the reach of the curette. Furthermore, curettage may contribute to infectious morbidity and therefore should be avoided.

Lesson 5 Do not give up too easily, but if you encounter blood, pus, or adhesions, do the procedure abdominally. Experience proved the feasibility of VTS in many cases not considered to qualify for this approach under the relative contraindications. Thus it appears appropriate for the operator willing to give the vaginal route a fair try to start the procedure per vaginam, but to alter the operative course upon failure to visualize or mobilize the fallopian tubes after a reasonably long exploration of the peritoneal cul-de-sac. Serendipity and acquired surgical skill probably account for our success in this circumstance. However, the corollary is also valid; if significant amounts (greater than 10 ml) of fluid, or blood or dense adhesions are encountered on entering the peritoneal cul-de-sac, or if attempted entry proves unusually difficult, mini-laparotomy or standard laparotomy is mandatory to ensure definitive management of the pelvic problem (total, bilateral salpingectomy, or more may be necessary).

Lesson 6 For optimal results, the surgeon should take into account the individual's clinical circumstances in choosing the method for sterilization. Based on this prospective study, we feel VTS is a viable (and underutilized) method of sterilization. It is a fortunate inevitability that surgeons gain skill in a given procedure according to their inclination and the opportunity to practice their art. Unfortunately, with facility comes the advocacy that "their" procedure is the best or the only way to solve the problem. It seems to us that, at this stage in the practice of sterilization procedures, there is *no universally applicable method* for all situations. The method best suited for an individual patient should be selected and the surgeon should use a triage concept in deciding which approach to take toward tubal sterilization. We have found the criteria shown in Table 12-2 to be of help in deciding the specific operation most suited to the individual patient.

The reader will note that, for the vast majority of women, tubal sterilization is optimally an outpatient procedure, performable by

Table 12-2
Outpatient Sterilization Selection Plan

Clinical Status	VTS	Mini-laparotomy	Laparoscopy	Inpatient Procedure (type)
Obese with slight pelvic relaxation	+ +	+	+	+ (Vaginal hysterectomy)
Extreme uterine retroversion but mobile	+ +	+	+	+ (Vaginal hysterectomy)
Immediately postabortal (less than 8 weeks)	+ +	+	+	...
Immediately postabortal (greater than 8 weeks but less than 12 weeks)	−	+ +	+	...
Postpartum (umbilical or suprafundal)	−	+ +	−	+ (Mini-laparotomy)
Palpable residue of PID and/or cul-de-sac adhesions	−	+ +	−	+ (Mini-laparotomy)
Thin and lax abdominal wall	+	+ +	+	...

Condition				
Deep vagina, high uterine suspension, and/or previous surgery	−	+ +	+	+ (Maxi-laparotomy)
Poor nutritional status (overweight or underweight)	+	+ +	+	...
Concomitant medical problems	−	−	−	+ (Mini-laparotomy)
Nulliparous with muscular or high uterine suspension	−	+	+ +	...
Extreme obesity with high uterine suspension	−	−	−	+ + (Maxi-laparotomy)
Obese with fibroids or other gynecologic pathology	−	−	−	+ + (Hysterectomy)

+ : Indicated
− : Contraindicated
+ + : Procedure of choice

VTS, mini-laparotomy, or laparoscopy. However, some patients merit in-hospital procedures, including hysterectomy or, in certain cases, no surgery at all. As with nonmedical aspects of life, the surgeon should resist the tendency to make the individual fit the mold and should adapt the treatment to fit the patient.

REFERENCES

1. Inman, WH: Thromboembolic disease and the steroidal content of oral contraceptives. A report to the Committee on Safety of Drugs. *Br Med J* 2:203, 1970.

2. Stolley PDJA: Thrombosis with low estrogen oral contraceptives. *Am J Epidemiol* 102:197, 1975.

3. Metropolitan Life Insurance Company Table of Weight Versus Height from Build and Blood Pressure Study, Society of Actuaries, 1959.

4. Brown HP, Schanzer SN: Vaginal tubal sterilization–lessons learned after 400 cases. Presented at Armed Forces District-American College of Obstetricians and Gynecologists 18th Annual Meeting, October 3, 1979.

EPILOGUE

In the preceding pages we have attempted to give the critical reader an overview of the presently available and popular methods of permanent female contraception. Our emphasis on the vaginal route is based on biases developed by weighing the advantages and disadvantages of all of these approaches. Having selected the vaginal route and the Kroener fimbriectomy as the method of choice, we became convinced by our experience of the merits of this technique and its applicability not only to the sophisticated, well-equipped, city hospital or facility, but also to the smaller rural hospitals here in the United States and elsewhere in the world. In the past ten years there has occurred a remarkable expansion in the field of family planning, of which permanent contraception by tubal sterilization is an important aspect, with roots in the work of pioneers in surgery as far back as 1850. Continued research and evaluation in this field can only lead to better techniques, greater refinement of methodology, and more benefits for the individual patient and mankind as a whole.

As family planners, our small participation in this endeavor has been most gratifying, particularly as it relates to the observable improvements in the quality of life of our patients and, hopefully, of the women of the rest of the world through easy, safe, and affordable reproductive security.

The following audiovisual aids have proven helpful in counseling the tubal sterilization candidate prior to the operative procedure:

CHARTS

1. The Female Reproductive System—Illustrations for Patient Counseling. Searle & Co., San Juan, Puerto Rico, 1976 (more suitable for individual counseling).
2. The Female Reproductive System. Ortho REACH Series, Ortho Pharmaceutical Co., Raritan, NJ, 1973 (more suitable for group counseling).

MODELS

The Ortho Model of the Internal Female Genitalia. Ortho Pharmaceutical Company. Raritan, NJ (useful for both group and individual counseling).

FILMS

1. Tubal Ligation. Ob-Gyn Series, #21. Milner-Fenwich Co. 2125 Green Spring Drive, Timonium, MD 21093, 8 mm, 16 mm, videocassette (discusses reproduction, explains how sterilization prevents conception, and describes the three techniques of sterilization).
2. Voluntary Tubal Sterilization. Professional Research, Inc., 461 North La Brea Ave., Los Angeles, CA, 90036 (contents similar to #1).

Massachusetts Medical Society

Authorized Consent Form

REQUEST FOR STERILIZATION

Patient _____ Age _____

                                                       A.M.

Date _____ Time _____ P.M. Place _____

I request Doctor _____ , and any assistants

of his choice, to perform upon _____
                                               (name of patient)

the following operation: _____
                                 (state nature and extent of operation)

It has been explained to me that this operation is intended to result in sterility although this result is not guaranteed. I understand that a sterile person is NOT capable of becoming a parent.

I voluntarily request the operation and understand that if it proves successful, the results will be permanent and it will thereafter be physically impossible for me to inseminate, or to conceive or bear children.

                           Signed _____
                                             (Patient)

                           Signed _____
                                             (Spouse)

Witness _____

PRE- & POSTOPERATIVE INSTRUCTIONS FOR PATIENTS
HAVING TUBAL LIGATION

Your surgery is scheduled for _____

Immediately after your clinic visit at Reproductive Services, go directly to Park North Hospital to have a chest x-ray.

THE NIGHT BEFORE SURGERY
1. Shampoo your hair and take a shower.
2. Remove all fingernail polish.
3. Take a mild laxative.
4. Do NOT eat or drink any food or liquid after 10 PM the night before surgery. It is VERY important that your stomach be completely empty.
5. Clip your pubic hair short - do not shave.

THE DAY OF THE SURGERY
1. Take a shower or tub bath before leaving home. Use an antibacterial soap like Safeguard or Dial.
2. Do not apply any make-up, particularly not eye make-up or lipstick.
3. Do not wear hairpins, earrings,-watches, jewelry, etc., of any kind to the hospital.
4. Long hair should be braided or secured with a rubber band at the base of your neck.
5. Give yourself an enema; a "Fleet" or "Enemeeze" Enema.
6. Take a sanitary belt from home to the hospital with you.
7. Do not worry if you happen to be having your menstrual period at the time of the surgery. This will not affect the procedure.
8. If you develop a cold, cough, sore throat or fever before the surgery, notify the clinic. In this case, the doctor may want to postpone the surgery. The clinic will consult the doctor about your condition.
9. Be at the admitting office at Park North General Hospital, 4330 Vance Jackson, at 6:30 AM. The phone number is 341-5131. IT IS ESSENTIAL THAT YOU ARRIVE ON TIME.

OTHER IMPORTANT INFORMATION
1. At the hospital you will need to remove any contact lenses, glasses, dentures and bridgework.
2. You will not be able to drive a car for 24 to 48 hours after the surgery. A responsible adult MUST be available to drive you home after the surgery.
3. No one will be angry if you decide not to have the surgery. This is a completely voluntary decision on your part. If you change your mind and decide not to have the surgery, let the clinic know in plenty of time so that another woman may be scheduled in your place.
4. You should avoid sexual relations for 2 to 4 weeks after the surgery.
5. After the surgery, call Reproductive Services to make your check up appointment.

PLEASE CALL REPRODUCTIVE SERVICES AT 826-6336 IF YOU HAVE A PROBLEM OR A QUESTION ABOUT THE SURGERY OR HOW YOU FEEL AFTERWARD.

Take the referral slip below with you to the hospital to have your chest x-ray.

— —

REPRODUCTIVE SERVICES, INC.
This is a referral for a chest x-ray for a patient requesting a tubal ligation.

NAME: _____ AGE: _____ TELEPHONE: _____

ADDRESS: _____ DATE OF PLANNED SURGERY: _____

DOCTOR: _____TITLE XX _____ PRIVATE INSURANCE _____ MEDICAID _____ OTHER ____

Chest x-ray is to be taken at Park North General Hospital, 4330 Vance Jackson, San Antonio, Texas; 341-5131.   Date: _____ between 8 am and 4 pm.

Slip made out by: _____ Date: _____

INDEX

Abortion, 3, 98. *See also* Luteal
pregnancy
Abscess, tubo-ovarian, 84, 85–88
Activities, postoperative, 43
Adenomyosis, and VTS, 86, 96
Adhesions, 97, 98
Age. *See* Minors
Ampicillin, 85
Anatomy
surgical, 74
utero-ovarian, 11
Anesthesia, 2, 96
administration of, 55–56
choice of, 53–54
complications,
incidence of, 84, 85
general, contraindications, 56
for laparoscopy, closed, 28–30
in method comparison, 20
for tubal ligation after vaginal
delivery, 35
with VTS, 8
Anesthesiologist, 19, 60
Antibiotics, 85, 87
Antiemesis, 79
Assistant, surgical, 19
Audiovisual aids, 40, 103

Banding, 10, 16–17
Bleeding, 9
incidence of, 84, 85
incisional, 88–89
patient questions, 44
Bleeding disorders, 96
Blood, 97
Blood vessel damage, 2
Bowel burns, 2, 9, 29

Cardiac monitoring, 56
Cellulitis, 86, 87
Cephalosporins, 85
Cesarean section, 8, 35
Clinical experience

complications, postoperative,
85–92
discussion of, 83–85
failure of sterilization, 89–90
granulation, persistent, 89
incisional bleeding, 88–89
lessons learned, 95–100
long-term follow-up, 92–93
menstrual timing for surgery,
90–92
pelvic inflammatory disease, 85
pelvic inflammatory disease
with tubo-ovarian abscess,
85–88
pelvic pain without PID, 88
Clipping, 10, 16, 17
Coagulation, endothermic, 27
Codeine sulfate, 79
Colpoceliotomy, 17
Colpotomy. *See* Vaginal tubal
sterilization
Complications, 2, 85
anesthesia-related, 56
of closed laparotomy, 29
in method comparison, 19
in mini-laparotomy, 31
physician discussion of, 40
of tubal sterilization, 2
with VTS, 9, 85–92
Consent, 40, 49, 50, 51, 52. *See
also* Failure, of sterilization
Consent form, 104
Constitutional factors, 87, 88
Contraception
alternative methods, 33–34
before surgery, 90
physician discussion of, 40
trends in methods, 3–5
Contraceptive failure, 48–50
Contraindications
for closed laparoscopy, 29
for general anesthesia, 56
for VTS, 96

107

Counseling, 38, 39–42, 103
Cramps, postoperative, 80. *See also*
　　Pain
Criminal liability, 50–51. *See also*
　　Medical-legal considerations
Culdotomy. *See* Vaginal tubular
　　sterilization
Cultural factors
　and anesthetic choice, 54
　and counseling, 39–40
Cyanomethacrylate plugs, 34

Diet, 79
Dilation and curettage (D&C), pre-
　　operative, 96–97
Discharge, of patient, 80
Discharge, vaginal, 80

Economic status, 39. *See also*
　　Federal regulations
Ectopic pregnancy, 21, 83, 90
Endotracheal intubation, 55
Equipment
　for laparoscopy, 7–8, 29
　in method comparison, 20
　for VTS, 8, 58–60
Eugenic sterilization, 48

Failure, of sterilization
　discussion of, 40
　ectopic pregnancy, 90
　luteal phase pregnancy, 91, 92
　methods comparison, 10
　postpartum procedures, 34
Federal regulations, 32, 39, 46, 49
Fentanyl citrate, 55
Ferric subsulfate, 89
Fever, postoperative, 80
Fimbriectomy, 10, 14. *See also*
　　Kroener procedure; Kroener
　　technique; Operative technique
Fistula formation, 9, 12, 89, 90
Follow-up, long-term, 92–93
Fulguration, 10, 16, 28, 29

Granulation, 44, 84, 85, 89

Hemorrhage, postoperative, 80
History evaluation, 38
Hormones, long-acting, 33–34.
　　See also Oral contraceptives
Hulka procedure, 28
Hysterectomy, 32, 46, 98, 99

Infection, signs of, 43–44. *See also*
　　Pelvic inflammatory disease
Inpatient procedures, 98–99. *See also*
　　Hysterectomy; Laparotomy
Instruments, for VTS, 58–60
Intrauterine devices (IUDs), 3, 4, 33
　patient questions, 45
　and postoperative infections, 85
　and VTS, 96
Irving procedure, 10, 14–15

Kroener procedure, 10, 11, 14, 69, 83,
　　84, 91. *See also* Clinical experi-
　　ence; Operative technique
Kroener technique
　choice of, 18
　fimbrial end amputation, 70
　surgical anatomy, 73
　tubal ligation, 71

Laboratory work, 38, 39, 58, 81
Laparoscopy
　choice of, 20
　clinical status and, 98–99
　closed, 27–30
　comparison of, 18–19
　open, 30
　vs VTS, 7–8
Laparotomies
　clinical status and, 98–99
　maxi-, 99
　mini-, 18–19, 31–32, 83, 84, 99
Legal considerations. *See* Medical-legal
　　considerations
Legislation, 49. *See also* Federal
　　regulations
Leiomyomata, and VTS, 96
Lidocaine, 55
Ligation procedures. *See* Methods,
　　choice of

110